MRI at a Glance

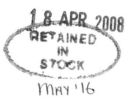

MRI at a Glance

CATHERINE WESTBROOK

MSc DCRR CTC

Director of Training and Education
Lodestone Patient Care Ltd

Blackwell
Science

© 2002 by Blackwell Science Ltd,
a Blackwell Publishing Company
Editorial Offices:
Osney Mead, Oxford OX2 0EL, UK
  Tel: +44 (0)1865 206206
Blackwell Science, Inc., 350 Main Street,
Malden, MA 02148-5018, USA
  Tel: +1 781 388 8250
Iowa State Press, a Blackwell Publishing
Company, 2121 State Avenue, Ames, Iowa
50014-8300, USA
  Tel: +1 515 292 0140
Blackwell Science Asia Pty, 54 University
Street, Carlton, Victoria 3053, Australia
  Tel: +61 (0)3 9347 0300
Blackwell Wissenschafts Verlag,
Kurfürstendamm 57, 10707 Berlin, Germany
  Tel: +49 (0)30 32 79 060

First published 2002 by Blackwell Science Ltd

Library of Congress Cataloging-in-Publication Data
is available

ISBN 0-632-05619-3

A catalogue record for this title is
available from the British Library

Set in 9 on 11.5 pt Times
by SNP Best-set Typesetter Ltd., Hong Kong
Printed and bound in Great Britain at
the Alden Press, Oxford and Northampton

For further information on
Blackwell Science, visit our website:
www.blackwell-science.com.

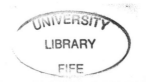

Contents

Preface

MRI at a Glance is one of a series of books that presents complex information on medical subjects in an easily accessible format. The aim is to have all information on a particular topic summarized on two facing pages of the book so that the reader has essential points at their fingertips. When the publishers approached me about including MRI in this format, I was rather sceptical. Could all relevant material, including text, diagrams and images be abbreviated and presented in a similar fashion to other books in the series? Being happy to try almost anything once, and fortified by my previous successful attempts at authorship, I decided to have a go!

MRI at a Glance aims to provide core knowledge on MRI theory in an accessible format. Information on a particular subject is mostly presented on a single page or double page format so that essential points can be instantly seen and understood. All topics from magnetism to safety, K space to pulse sequences, image contrast to artefacts are included using short bulleted text linked to key diagrams, tables and images. A glossary of common terms and appendices on acronyms and artefacts are also included. The main uses for this type of book as opposed to longer texts are for revision purposes and where fuller explanations are too daunting. Despite the concise nature of the material and the inevitable omission of some of the more complicated issues, I believe that this book fulfills its purpose and will support the education of clinical practitioners in the glorious art and science of MRI.

Acknowledgements

In my previous books, I lauded the praises of 'the worlds most perfect children', Adam, Ben and Madeleine. This time I do so again, but also thank them from the bottom of my heart for their unconditional love and support. This gratitude is also extended to my friends and family for not being my judge and jury, but for being there when I needed them.

This book is dedicated to Francina Sip, a magnificent woman who filled the space in my life and made me complete.

Glossary

2D volumetric acquisition — acquisition where a small amount of data is acquired from each slice before repeating the TR

3D volumetric acquisition — acquisition where the whole imaging volume is excited so that the images can be viewed in any plane

actual TE — the time between the echo and the next RF pulse in SSFP

aliasing — artefact produced when anatomy outside the FOV is mismapped inside the FOV

alignment — when nuclei are placed in an external magnetic field their magnetic moments line up with the magnetic field flux lines

Alnico — alloy that is used to make permanent magnets

Ampere's law — determines the magnitude and direction of the magnetic field due to a current; if you point your right hand thumb along the direction of the current, then the magnetic field points along the direction of the curled fingers

angular momentum — the spin of MR active nuclei that depends on the balance between the number of protons and neutrons in the nucleus

anti-parallel alignment — describes the alignment of magnetic moments in the opposite direction to the main field

atomic number — sum of protons in the nucleus

B_0 — the main magnetic field measured in tesla

bipolar — describes a magnet with two poles, north and south

black blood imaging — acquisitions in which blood vessels are black

blood oxygen level dependent (BOLD) — a functional MRI technique that uses the differences in magnetic susceptibility between oxyhaemoglobin and de-oxyhaemoglobin to image areas of activated cerebral cortex

bright blood imaging — acquisitions in which blood vessels are bright

Brownian motion — internal motion of the molecules

central lines — area of K space filled with the shallowest phase encoding slopes

classical theory — uses the direction of the magnetic moments to illustrate alignment

chemical misregistration — artefact along the phase axis caused by the phase difference between fat and water

chemical shift — artefact along the frequency axis caused by the frequency difference between fat and water

co-current flow — flow in the same direction as slice excitation

contrast to noise ratio (CNR) — difference in SNR between two points

counter-current flow — flow in the opposite direction to slice excitation

cross excitation — energy given to nuclei in adjacent slices by the RF pulse

cross talk — energy given to nuclei in adjacent slices due to spin lattice relaxation

cryogen bath — area around the coils of wire in which cryogens are placed

cryogens — substances used to supercool the coils of wire in a superconducting magnet

coherent — the magnetic moments of hydrogen are at the same place on the precessional path

decay — loss of transverse magnetization

dephasing — the magnetic moments of hydrogen are at a different place on their precessional path

diamagnetism — property that shows a small magnetic moment that opposes the applied field

diffusion — a term used to describe moving molecules due to random thermal motion

echo spacing — spacing between each echo in FSE

echo train — series of 180° rephasing pulse and echoes in a fast spin echo pulse sequence

echo train length (ETL) or turbo factor — the number of 180° RF pulses and resultant echoes in FSE

effective TE — the time between the echo and the RF pulse that initiated it in SSFP and FSE sequences

electrons — orbit the nucleus in distinct shells and are negatively charged

emf — drives a current in a circuit and is the result of a changing magnetic field inducing an electric field

entry slice phenomena — contrast difference of flowing nuclei relative to the stationary nuclei because they are fresh

even echo rephasing — the use of evenly spaced echoes to reduce artefact

excitation — the energy transfer from the RF pulse to the NMV

extrinsic contrast parameters — contrast parameters that are controlled by the system operator

fast Fourier transform (FFT)	mathematical conversion of frequency/time domain to frequency/amplitude
ferromagnetism	property of a substance that ensures that it remains magnetic, is permanently magnetized and subsequently becomes a permanent magnet
field of view (FOV)	area of anatomy covered in an image
FLAIR (fluid attenuated inversion recovery)	IR sequences that nulls the signal from CSF
flip angle	the angle of the NMV to B_0
flow encoding axes	axes along which bipolar gradients act in order to sensitize flow along the axis of the gradient; used in phase contrast MRA
flow phenomena	artefacts produced by flowing nuclei
flow related enhancement	decrease in time of flight due to a decrease in velocity of flow
free induction decay (FID)	loss of signal due to relaxation
frequency encoding	locating a signal according to its frequency
fresh spins	nuclei that have not been beaten down by repeated RF pulses
fringe field	stray magnetic field outside the bore of the magnet
functional MR imaging (fMRI)	a rapid MR imaging technique that acquires images of the brain during activity or stimulus and at rest
ghosting	motion artefact in the phase axis
gradient amplifier	supplies power to the gradient coils
gradient echo pulse sequence	one that uses a gradient to regenerate an echo
gradient echo	echo produced as a result of gradient rephasing
gradient spoiling	the use of gradients to dephase magnetic moments; the opposite of rewinding
gradients	coils of wire that alter the magnetic field strength in a linear fashion when a current is passed through them
gyro-magnetic ratio	the precessional frequency of an element at 1.0 T
high velocity signal loss	increase in time of flight due to an increase in the velocity of flow
homogeneity	the evenness of the magnetic field
hybrid sequences	combination of FSE and EPI sequences where a series of gradient echoes are interspersed with spin echoes. In this way susceptibility artefacts are reduced
incoherent	means that the magnetic moments of hydrogen are at different places on the precessional path
in-flow effect	another term for entry slice phenomenon
inhomogeneities	areas where the magnetic field strength is not exactly the same as the main field strength
intra-voxel dephasing	phase difference between flow and stationary nuclei in a voxel
intrinsic contrast mechanisms	contrast parameters that do not come under the operators control
ions	atoms with an excess or deficit of electrons
isotopes	atoms of the same element having a different mass number
J coupling	a process that describes the reduction the spin spin interactions in fat, thereby increasing its T2 decay time
K space	an area where raw data is stored
Larmor equation	used to calculate the frequency or speed of precession for a specific nucleus in a specific magnetic field strength
Lenz's law	law that states induced emf is in a direction so that it opposes the change in magnetic field which causes it
longitudinal plane	the axis parallel to B_0
magnetic flux density	number of flux lines per unit area
magnetic isocentre	the centre of the bore of the magnet in all planes
magnetic moment	denotes the direction of the north/south axis of a magnet and the amplitude of the magnetic field
magnetic lines of flux	lines of force running from the magnetic south to the north poles of the magnet
magnetic susceptibility	ability of a substance to become magnetized
magnetism	a property of all matter that depends on the magnetic susceptibility of the atom
magnitude image	unsubtracted image combination of flow sensitized data
mass number	sum of neutrons and protons in the nucleus
MR active	nuclei that possess an odd number of protons
MR angiography	method of visualizing vessels that contain flowing nuclei by producing a contrast between them and the stationary nuclei
MR signal	the voltage induced in the receiver coil
net magnetization vector (NMV)	the magnetic vector produced as a result of the alignment of excess hydrogen nuclei with B_0
neutrons	particles in the nucleus that have no charge
number of signal averages	the number of times an echo is encoded with the same slope of phase encoding gradient
Nyquist theorem	states that a frequency must be sampled at at least twice the

outer lines — highest frequency in the echo in order to reproduce it reliably

outer lines area of K space filled with the steepest phase encoding gradient slopes

parallel alignment describes the alignment of magnetic moments in the same direction as the main field

paramagnetism property whereby substances affect external magnetic fields in a positive way, resulting in a local increase in the magnetic field

partial averaging filling only a proportion of K space with data and putting zeroes in the remainder

partial echo sampling only part of the echo and extrapolating the remainder in K space

perfusion a measure of the quality of vascular supply to a tissue

permanent magnets magnets that retain their magnetism

phase contrast angiography technique that generates vascular contrast by applying a bipolar gradient to stationary and moving spins thereby changing their phase

phase encoding locating a signal according to its phase

phase image subtracted image combination of flow sensitized data

phase the position of a magnetic moment on its precessional path at any given time

polarity the direction of a gradient, i.e. which end is greater than B_0 and which is lower than B_0. Depends on the direction of the current through the gradient coil

precession the secondary spin of magnetic moments around B_0

protons particles in the nucleus that are positively charged

proton density the number of protons in a unit volume of tissue

proton density weighting image that demonstrates the differences in the proton densities of the tissues

pulse control unit co-ordinates the switching on and off of the gradient and RF transmitter coils at appropriate times during the pulse sequence

pulse sequence a series of RF pulses, gradients applications and intervening time periods; used to control contrast

quantum theory uses the energy level of the nuclei to illustrate alignment

quenching process by which there is a sudden loss of the superconductivity of the magnet coils so that the magnet becomes resistive

ramp sampling where sampling data points are collected when the gradient rise time is almost complete. Sampling occurs while the gradient is still reaching maximum amplitude, while the gradient is at maximum amplitude and as it begins to decline

readout gradient the frequency encoding gradient

receive bandwidth range of frequencies that are sampled during readout

recovery growth of longitudinal magnetization

relaxation process by which hydrogen loses energy

repetition time (TR) time between each excitation pulse

rephasing creating in-phase magnetization, usually by using an RF pulse or a gradient

residual transverse magnetization transverse magnetization left over from previous RF pulses in steady state conditions

resistive magnet an electromagnet created by passing current through loops of wire

resonance an energy transition that occurs when an object is subjected to a frequency the same as its own

rewinding the use of a gradient to rephase magnetic moments

RF amplifier supplies power to the RF transmitter coils

RF pulse short burst of RF energy which excites nuclei into a high energy state

RF spoiling the use of digitized RF to transmit and receive at a certain phase

RF transmitter coil coil that transmits RF at the resonant frequency of hydrogen to excite nuclei and move them into a high energy state

rise time the time it takes a gradient to switch on, achieve the required gradient slope, and switch off again

sampling rate rate at which samples are taken during readout

sampling time the time that the readout gradient is switched on for

saturation occurs when the NMV is flipped to a full 180°

sequential acquisition acquisition where all the data from each slice are acquired before going on to the next

shim coil extra coils used to make the magnetic field as homogeneous as possible

shimming process whereby the evenness of the magnetic filed is optimized

signal-to-noise ratio (SNR) ratio of signal relative to noise

single shot a sequence where all the lines of K

	space are acquired during a single TR period	T1 recovery	growth of longitudinal magnetization as a result of spin lattice relaxation
slice encoding	the separation of individual slice locations by phase in volume acquisitions	T1 time	time taken for 63% of the longitudinal magnetization to recover
slice selection	selecting a slice using a gradient	T1 weighted image	image that demonstrates the differences in the T1 times of the tissues
spatial encoding	spatially locating a signal in three dimensions	T2 decay	loss of transverse magnetization as a result of spin–spin relaxation
spatial resolution	the ability to distinguish two points as separate	T2 time	time taken for 63% of the transverse magnetization to decay
spectroscopy	provides a frequency spectrum of a given tissue based on the molecular and chemical structures of that tissue	T2 weighted image	image that demonstrates the differences in the T2 times of the tissues
spin down	the population of high energy hydrogen nuclei that align their magnetic moments antiparallel to the main field	T2*	dephasing due to magnetic field inhomogeneities
spin echo pulse sequence	one that uses a 180° rephasing pulse to generate an echo	TI	time from inversion; a parameter used in IR sequences
spin echo	echo produced as a result of a 180° rephasing pulse	time of flight angiography	technique that generates vascular contrast by utilizing the in-flow effect
spin lattice relaxation	process by which energy is given up to the surrounding lattice	time of flight	rate of flow in a given time. Causes some flowing nuclei to receive one RF pulse only and therefore produce a signal void
spin–spin relaxation	process by which interactions between the magnetic fields of adjacent nuclei causes dephasing	time to echo TE	time between the excitation pulse and the echo
spin up	the population of low energy hydrogen nuclei that align their magnetic moments parallel to B_0	transceiver	coil that both transmits RF and receives the MR signal
spoiling	a process of dephasing spins either with a gradient or an RF pulse	transmit bandwidth	range of frequencies transmitted in an RF pulse
steady state	a situation when the TR is shorter than both the T1 and T2 relaxation times of all the tissues	transverse plane	the axis perpendicular to B_0
		turbo factor or echo train length	the number of 180° rephasing pulse/echoes/phase encodings per TR in fast spin echo
stimulated-echo acquisition mode (STEAM)	spatial localization technique used in spectroscopy	volume coil	coil that transmits and receives signal over a large volume of the patient
STIR (short TI inversion recovery)	sequence used to suppress fat	voxel volume	volume of tissue in the patient
superconducting magnet	electromagnet that use supercooled coils of wire so that there is no inherent resistance in the system. The current flows, and therefore the magnetism is generated without a driving voltage	watergrams	FSE sequence using very long TRs, TEs and ETLs to produce very heavy T2 weighting

1 Magnetism and electromagnetism

Magnetic susceptibility

The **magnetic susceptibility** of a substance is the ability of external magnetic fields to affect the nuclei of a particular atom, and is related to the electron configurations of that atom. The nucleus of an atom, which is surrounded by paired electrons, is more protected from, and unaffected by, the external magnetic field than the nucleus of an atom with unpaired electrons. There are three types of magnetic susceptibility: **paramagnetism**, **diamagnetism** and **ferromagnetism**.

Paramagnetism

Paramagnetic substances contain unpaired electrons within the atom that induce a small magnetic field about themselves known as the **magnetic moment**. With no external magnetic field these magnetic moments occur in a random pattern and cancel each other out. In the presence of an external magnetic field, paramagnetic substances align with the direction of the field and so the magnetic moments add together. Paramagnetic substances affect external magnetic fields in a positive way, resulting in a local increase in the magnetic field (Fig. 1.1). An example of a paramagnetic substance is oxygen.

Diamagnetism

With no external magnetic field present, diamagnetic substances show no net magnetic moment as the electron currents caused by their motions add to zero. When an external magnetic field is applied, diamagnetic substances show a small magnetic moment that opposes the applied field (Fig. 1.2). Substances of this type are therefore slightly repelled by the magnetic field and have negative magnetic susceptibilities. Examples of diamagnetic substances include water and inert gases.

Ferromagnetism

When a ferromagnetic substance comes into contact with a magnetic field, the results are strong attraction and alignment. It retains its magnetization even when the external magnetic field has been removed (Fig. 1.3). Ferromagnetic substances remain magnetic, are permanently magnetized and subsequently become permanent magnets. An example of a ferromagnetic substance is iron.

Magnets are **bipolar** as they have two poles, north and south. The magnetic field exerted by them produces magnetic field lines or lines of force running from the magnetic south to the north poles of the magnet. They are called **magnetic lines of flux** (Fig. 1.4). The number of lines per unit area is called the **magnetic flux density**. The strength of the magnetic field, expressed by the notation (B), (or in the case of more than one field, the primary field (B_0) and the secondary field (B_1), is measured in one of three units; **gauss (G)**, **kilogauss (kG)** and **tesla (T)**. If two magnets are brought close together, there are forces of attraction and repulsion between them depending on the orientation of their poles relative to each other. Like poles repel and opposite poles attract.

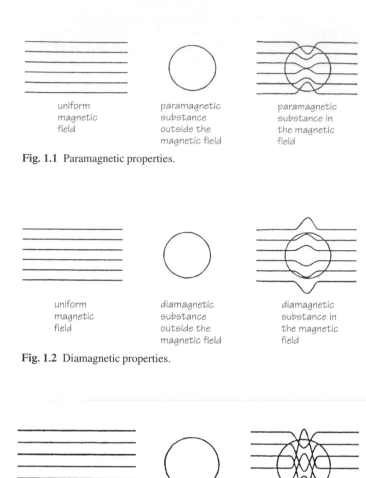

uniform magnetic field   paramagnetic substance outside the magnetic field   paramagnetic substance in the magnetic field

Fig. 1.1 Paramagnetic properties.

uniform magnetic field   diamagnetic substance outside the magnetic field   diamagnetic substance in the magnetic field

Fig. 1.2 Diamagnetic properties.

uniform magnetic field   ferromagnetic substance outside the magnetic field   ferromagnetic substance in the magnetic field

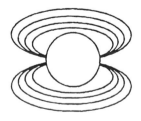

ferromagnetic substance after exposure to the magnetic field

Fig. 1.3 Ferromagnetic properties.

Electromagnetism

Magnetic fields are generated by moving charges (electrical current) (Fig. 1.5). The direction of the magnetic field can either be clockwise or counter-clockwise with respect to the direction of flow of the current. **Ampere's law** or **Fleming's Right hand rule** determines the magnitude and direction of the magnetic field due to a current; if you point your right hand thumb along the direction of the current, then the magnetic field points along the direction of the curled fingers.

Just as moving electrical charge generates magnetic fields, changing magnetic fields generate electric currents. When a magnet is moved in and out of a closed circuit, an oscillating current is produced which ceases the moment the magnet stops moving. Such a current is called an **induced electric current**.

Faraday's law of induction explains the phenomenon of an induced current. The change of magnetic flux through a closed circuit induces an **electromotive force (emf)** in the circuit. The emf drives a current in the circuit and is the result of a changing magnetic field inducing an electric field.

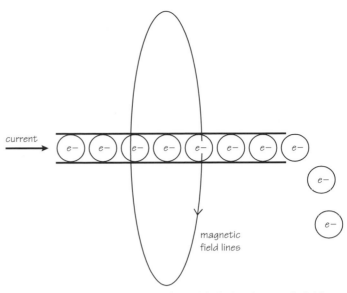

Fig. 1.5 Flow of electrons along a wire and the induced magnetic field.

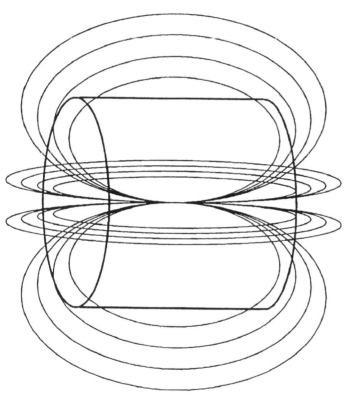

Fig. 1.4 Magnetic flux line.

The laws of electromagnetic induction state that the induced emf:
• is proportional to the rate of change of magnetic field and the area of the circuit;
• is in a direction so that it opposes the change in magnetic field which causes it (**Lenz's law**).

Electromagnetic induction is a basic physical phenomenon of MRI but is specifically involved in the following.
• The spinning charge of a hydrogen proton causes a magnetic field to be induced around it (see Chapter 2).
• The movement of the **net magnetization vector (NMV)** across the area of a receiver coil induces an electrical charge in the coil (see Chapter 4).

2 Atomic structure

The atom consists of the following particles (Fig. 2.1).

Protons
• These are in the nucleus.
• They are positively charged.

Neutrons
• These are in the nucleus.
• They have no charge.

Electrons
• These orbit the nucleus in distinct shells.
• They are negatively charged.

The following terms are used to characterize an atom.

Atomic number is the number of protons in the nucleus; it determines the type of element the atoms make up.

Mass number is the sum of the neutrons and protons in the nucleus.

Atoms of the same element having a different mass number are called **isotopes**.

In a stable atom the number of negatively charged electrons equals the number of positively charged protons. Atoms with a deficit or excess number of electrons are called **ions**.

Motion within the atom (Fig. 2.2)
• Negatively charged electrons spin on their own axis.
• Negatively charged electrons orbit the nucleus.
• The nucleus spins on its own axis.

Each type of motion produces a magnetic field (see Chapter 1). In MR we are concerned with the motion of the nucleus.

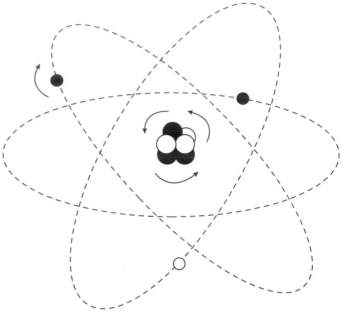

Fig. 2.2 Motion of particles in the atom.

MR active nuclei

Protons and neutrons spin about their own axes within the nucleus. The direction of spin is random so that some particles spin clockwise, and others anticlockwise.

• When a nucleus has an **even mass number** the spins cancel each other out so the nucleus has **no net spin**.

• When a nucleus has an **odd mass number**, the spins do not cancel each other out and the **nucleus spins**.

As protons have charge, a nucleus with an odd mass number has a net charge as well as a net spin. Owing to the laws of electromagnetic induction (see Chapter 1), a moving unbalanced charge induces a magnetic field around itself. The direction and size of the magnetic field is denoted by a magnetic moment or arrow (Fig. 2.3). The total magnetic moment of the nucleus is the vector sum of all the magnetic moments of protons in the nucleus. The length of the arrow represents the magnitude of the magnetic moment. The direction of the arrow denotes the direction of alignment of the magnetic moment.

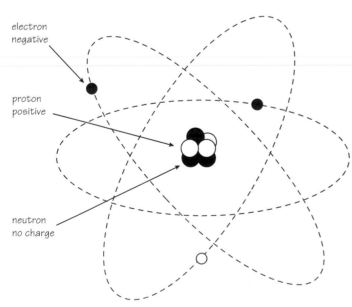

electron
negative

proton
positive

neutron
no charge

Fig. 2.1 The atom.

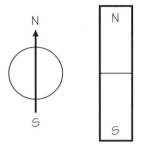

Fig. 2.3 The magnetic moment of the hydrogen nucleus.

Nuclei with an odd number of protons are said to be **MR active**. They act like tiny bar magnets. There are many types of elements that are MR active. They all have odd mass numbers. They are:

Hydrogen 1,　Carbon 13,　Fluorine 19,　Phosphorous 31,
Nitrogen 15,　Oxygen 17,　Sodium 23.

The **hydrogen nucleus** is the MR active nucleus used in MRI. This nucleus consists of a single proton (atomic number 1). It is used for MR imaging because:

- it is abundant in the human body (e.g. in fat and water);
- its solitary proton gives it a large magnetic moment.

3 Alignment and precession

Alignment

In a normal environment the magnetic moments of MR active nuclei point in a random direction, thus they produce no overall magnetic effect. When nuclei are placed in an external magnetic field their magnetic moments line up with the magnetic field flux lines. This is called **alignment** (Fig. 3.1). Alignment can be described using two theories: the classical theory and the quantum theory.

The classical theory

This uses the direction of the magnetic moments to illustrate alignment (Fig. 3.2).
• **Parallel alignment** describes the alignment of magnetic moments in the **same** direction as the main field.
• **Anti-parallel alignment** describes the alignment of magnetic moments in the **opposite** direction to the main field.

At room temperature there are always more nuclei with their magnetic moments aligned parallel to the main field than aligned antiparallel. The net magnetism of the patient (termed the **net magnetization vector** or **NMV**), which reflects the balance between the parallel and antiparallel magnetic moments, is therefore aligned parallel to the main field at room temperature (thermal equilibrium).

The quantum theory

This uses the energy level of the nuclei to illustrate alignment. There are certain factors that determine whether the magnetic moment of a nucleus aligns in the parallel direction or the antiparallel direction.

These are:
• the magnitude or strength of the external magnetic field, termed B_0 and measured in tesla (T);
• the energy level of the nucleus.

According to the quantum theory the magnetic moments of hydrogen nuclei align in the presence of an external magnetic field in the following two energy states or populations (Fig. 3.3).
• **Spin up** nuclei have low energy and do not have enough energy to oppose the main field. These are the nuclei that align their magnetic moments parallel to the main field in the classical description.
• **Spin down** nuclei have high energy and have enough energy to oppose the main field. These are the nuclei that align their magnetic moments antiparallel to the main field in the classical description.

The magnetic moments of the nuclei actually align at an angle to B_0 due to the force of repulsion between B_0 and the magnetic moments.

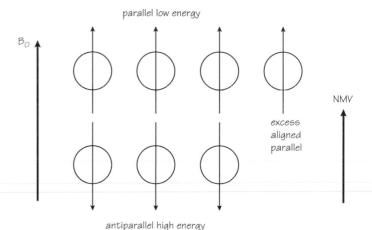

parallel low energy

B_0

NMV

excess aligned parallel

antiparallel high energy

Fig. 3.2 Alignment: the classical theory.

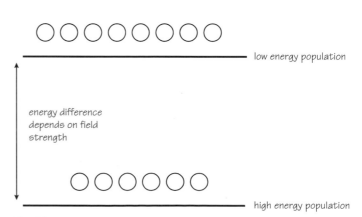

low energy population

energy difference depends on field strength

high energy population

Fig. 3.3 Alignment: the quantum theory.

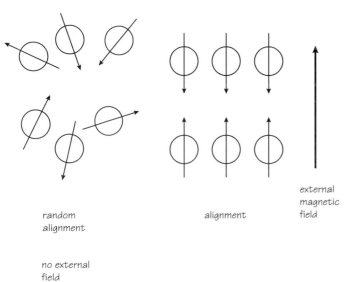

random alignment

alignment

external magnetic field

no external field

Fig. 3.1 Alignment.

What do the quantum and classical theories tell us?

• Hydrogen can only have two energy states – high or low. Therefore the magnetic moments of hydrogen can only align in the parallel or antiparallel directions. **The magnetic moments of hydrogen cannot orientate themselves in any other direction.**

• The temperature of the sample being imaged is an important factor that determines whether a nucleus is in the high or low energy population. In clinical imaging we discount thermal effects as we assume our patients are more or less the same temperature.

• The magnetic moments of hydrogen are constantly changing their orientation because nuclei are constantly moving between high and low energy states. The nuclei gain and lose energy from B_0 and their magnetic moments are constantly altering their alignment relative to B_0.

• At any one moment in time there are a greater proportion of nuclei with their magnetic moments aligned with the field than against it. This excess aligned with B_0 produces a net magnetic effect called the NMV which aligns with the main magnetic field.

• As the magnitude of the external magnetic field increases, more of the magnetic moments of the nuclei line up in the parallel direction because the amount of energy they must possess to oppose the field and line up antiparallel to the stronger magnetic field is increased. As the field strength increases, the low energy population increases and the high energy population decreases. As a result the NMV gets larger.

Precession

Every MR active nucleus is spinning on its own axis. Owing to the influence of the external magnetic field these nuclei produce a secondary spin or **spin wobble**.

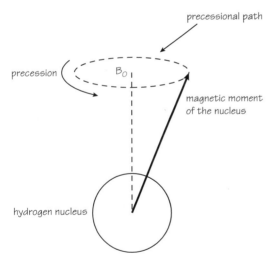

Fig. 3.4 Precession.

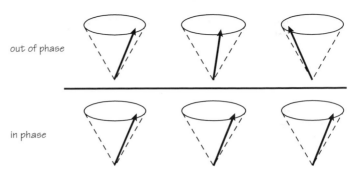

Fig. 3.5 Phase of magnetic moments around their precessional path.

This wobble is called **precession** and causes the magnetic moments of MR active nuclei to describe a circular path around B_0 (Fig. 3.4). The speed at which the magnetic moments wobble about the external magnetic field is called the **precessional frequency**.

The Larmor equation is used to calculate the frequency or speed of precession for a specific nucleus in a specific magnetic field strength. The Larmor equation is stated as follows.

$$\omega_0 = B_0 \times \gamma$$

where the precessional frequency is denoted by ω_0,

the strength of the external magnetic field is expressed in tesla and denoted by the symbol B_0,

the **gyromagnetic ratio** is the precessional frequency of a specific nucleus at 1 T and therefore has units of MHz/T. It is denoted by the symbol γ. As it is a constant of proportionality the precessional frequency is proportional to the strength of the external magnetic field.

The precessional frequencies of hydrogen (gyromagnetic ratio 42.57 MHz/T) commonly found in clinical MRI are:

• 21.285 MHz at 0.5 T,
• 42.57 MHz at 1 T,
• 63.86 MHz at 1.5 T.

The precessional frequency corresponds to the range of frequencies in the electromagnetic spectrum of **radiowaves**. Therefore hydrogen precesses at a low frequency and energy. At equilibrium the magnetic moments of the nuclei are out of phase with each other. Phase refers to the position of the magnetic moments on their circular precessional path (Fig. 3.5).

• **Out of phase** or **incoherent** means that the magnetic moments of hydrogen are at different places on the precessional path.

• **In phase** or **coherent** means that the magnetic moments of hydrogen are at the same place on the precessional path.

4 Resonance and signal generation

Resonance

Resonance is an energy transition that occurs when an object is subjected to a frequency the same as its own. In MR, resonance is induced by applying a **radiofrequency (RF) pulse**:
- at the same frequency as the precessing hydrogen nuclei;
- at 90° to B_0.

This causes the hydrogen nuclei to resonate (receive energy from the RF pulse) whereas other MR active nuclei do not resonate because their gyromagnetic ratios are different from that of hydrogen. Owing to the Larmor equation their precessional frequency is different and therefore they only resonate if RF at their specific precessional frequency is applied.

Two things happen at resonance: energy absorption and phase coherence.

Energy absorption

The hydrogen nuclei absorb energy from the RF pulse (excitation pulse) (Fig. 4.1). The absorption of applied RF energy at 90° to B_0 causes an increase in the number of high energy, spin up nuclei. If just the right amount of energy is applied the number of nuclei in the spin up position equals the number in the spin down position. As a result the NMV (which represents the balance between spin up and spin down nuclei) lies in the transverse plane as the net magnetization lies between the two energy states. As the NMV has been moved through 90° from B_0, it has a **flip or tip angle** of 90° (Fig. 4.2).

Phase coherence

The magnetic moments of the nuclei move into phase with each other.

As the magnetic moments are in phase both in the spin up and spin down positions and the spin up nuclei are in phase with the spin down nuclei, the net effect is one of precession so the NMV precesses in the transverse plane at the Larmor frequency.

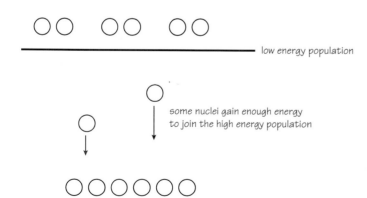

Fig. 4.1 Energy transfer during excitation.

Learning point
It is important to understand that when a patient is placed in the magnet and is scanned hydrogen nuclei do not move. Nuclei are not flipped onto their sides in the transverse plane and neither are their magnetic moments. Only the magnetic moments of the nuclei move, either aligning with or against B_0. This is because hydrogen can have only two energy states, high or low. It is the NMV that lies in the transverse plane not the magnetic moments, nor the nuclei themselves.

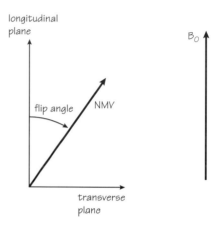

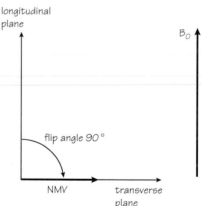

Fig. 4.2 The flip angle. What flip angle will give the maximum transverse magnetization?

The MR signal

A receiver coil is situated in the transverse plane (Fig. 4.3). As the NMV rotates around the transverse plane as a result of resonance, it passes across the receiver coil inducing a voltage in it. This voltage is the **MR signal**.

After a short period of time the RF pulse is removed. The signal induced in the receiver coil begins to decrease. This is because the in phase component of the NMV in the transverse plane, which is passing across the receiver coil, begins to decrease. The amplitude of the voltage induced in the receiver coil therefore decreases. This is called **free induction decay** (**FID**):

• 'free' because of the absence of the RF pulse; and

• 'induction decay' because of the decay of the induced signal in the receiver coil.

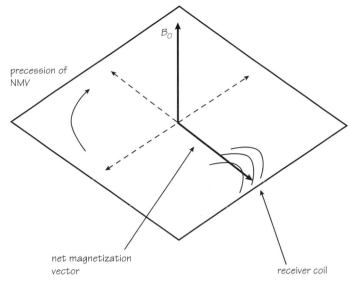

Fig. 4.3 Why would you expect the MR signal to be alternating?

5 Contrast mechanisms

What is contrast?

An image has contrast if there are areas of high signal (white on the image), as well as areas of low signal (dark on the image). Some areas have an intermediate signal (shades of grey in-between white and black). The NMV can be separated into the individual vectors of the tissues present in the patient such as fat, cerebro-spinal fluid (CSF) and muscle.

A tissue has a **high signal (white)** if it has a **large transverse component of magnetization**. If there is a large component of transverse magnetization, the amplitude of the magnetization received by the coil is large, and the signal induced in the coil is also large.

A tissue gives a **low signal (black)**, if it has a **small transverse component of magnetization**. If there is a small component of transverse magnetization, the amplitude of the magnetization received by the coil is small, and the signal induced in the coil is also small.

A tissue gives an **intermediate signal (grey)**, if it has a medium **transverse component of magnetization** (Fig. 5.1).

Image contrast is controlled by **extrinsic contrast parameters** (those that are controlled by the system operator). These include the following.

- **Repetition time (TR).** This is the time from the application of one RF pulse to the application of the next. It is measured in milliseconds (ms). The TR affects the length of a relaxation period after the application of one RF excitation pulse to the beginning of the next (Fig. 5.2).
- **Echo time (TE).** This is the time between an RF excitation pulse and the collection of the signal. The TE affects the length of the relaxation period after the removal of an RF excitation pulse and the peak of the signal received in the receiver coil. It is also measured in ms (Fig. 5.2).
- **Flip angle.** This is the angle through which the NMV is moved as a result of a RF excitation pulse.
- **Turbo-factor or echo train length (ETL/TF)** (*see* Chapter 13).
- **Time from inversion (TI).** (*see* Chapter 14).
- **'b' value** (*see* Chapter 20).

Image contrast is also controlled by **intrinsic contrast mechanisms** (those that do not come under the operators control). These include:

- **T1 recovery**
- **T2 decay**
- **proton density**
- **flow**
- **apparent diffusion coefficient (ADC).**

The composition of fat and water

All substances possess molecules that are constantly in motion. This molecular motion is made up of rotational and transitional movements. The faster the molecular motion, the more difficult it is for a substance to release energy to its surroundings.

- **Fat** comprises hydrogen atoms linked to carbon that make up large molecules. The large molecules in fat have a slow rate of molecular motion due to inertia of the large molecules. They also have a low inherent energy which means they are able to absorb energy efficiently.
- **Water** comprises hydrogen atoms linked to oxygen. It consists of small molecules with little inertia that have a high rate of molecular

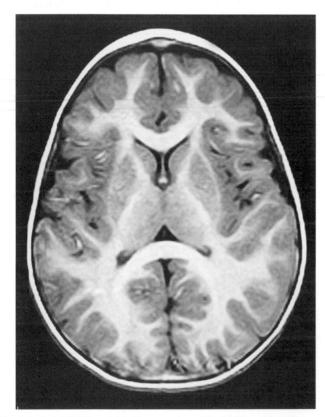

Fig. 5.1 Axial IR T1 weighted image using a TI of 700 ms. Note the exquisite contrast between grey and white matter.

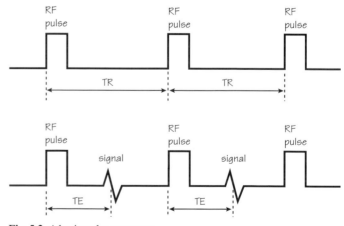

Fig. 5.2 A basic pulse sequence.

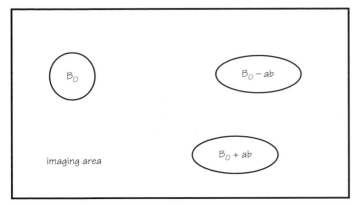

Fig. 5.3 Magnetic field inhomogeneities (ab represents these areas).

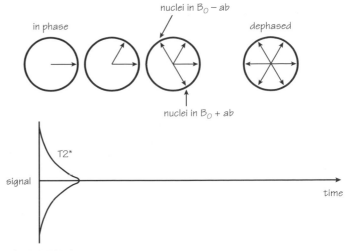

Fig. 5.4 T2* decay.

motion. They have a high inherent energy which means they are not able to absorb energy efficiently.

Because of these differences, tissues that contain fat and water produce different image contrast. This is because there are different relaxation rates in each tissue.

Relaxation processes

After the RF excitation pulse has been applied and resonance and the desired flip angle achieved, the RF pulse is removed. The signal induced in the receiver coil begins to decrease. This is because the coherent component of NMV in the transverse plane, which is passing across the receiver coil, begins to decrease. The amplitude of the voltage induced in the receiver coil therefore decreases. This is called **free induction decay (FID)**. The NMV in the transverse plane decreases due to **relaxation processes** and **field inhomogeneities**. The magnetization in each tissue relaxes at different rates. This is one of the factors that create image contrast.

The withdrawal of the RF produces several effects.
• Nuclei emit energy absorbed from the RF pulse through a process known as **spin lattice energy transfer** and shift their magnetic moments from the high energy state to the low energy state. The NMV recovers and realigns to B_0. This relaxation process is called **T1 recovery**.
• Nuclei lose precessional coherence or dephase and the NMV decays in the transverse plane. The dephasing relaxation process is called **T2 decay**.

Nuclei lose their coherence in two ways:
• by the interactions of the intrinsic magnetic fields of adjacent nuclei (**spin–spin energy transfer**); and
• by the **inhomogeneities** of the external magnetic field.

Despite attempts to make the main magnetic field as uniform as possible, inhomogeneities of the external magnetic field (Fig. 5.3) are inevitable and slightly alter the magnitude of B_0, i.e. some small areas of the field have a magnetic field strength of slightly more or less than the main field strength.

Owing to the Larmor equation, the precessional frequency of a spin is proportional to B_0. Spins that pass through these inhomogeneities experience magnetic field strengths that are slightly different from B_0 and their precessional frequencies change. This results in a change in their phase and dephasing of the NMV. Owing to a loss in phase coherence, transverse magnetization decays. This decay occurs exponentially and is known as **T2*** (Fig. 5.4). Magnetic field inhomogeneities cause the NMV to dephase before the intrinsic magnetic fields of nuclei can influence dephasing, i.e. T2* happens before T2. In order to produce images where T2 contrast can be visualized, there must be a mechanism to rephase spins and compensate for magnetic field inhomogeneities. This is done by using **pulse sequences**.

6 T1 recovery

T1 recovery is caused by the exchange of energy from nuclei to their surrounding environment or lattice. It is called **spin lattice energy transfer**. As the nuclei dissipate their energy their magnetic moments relax or return to B_0, i.e. they regain their longitudinal magnetization. The rate at which this occurs is an exponential process and it occurs at different rates in different tissues.

The **T1 time** of a particular tissue is an intrinsic contrast parameter that is inherent to the tissue being imaged. It is defined as the time it takes for 63% of the longitudinal magnetization to recover. The period of time during which this occurs is the time between one excitation pulse and the next or the **TR**. The TR therefore determines how much T1 recovery occurs in a particular tissue (Fig. 6.1).

T1 recovery in fat
• T1 relaxation occurs as a result of nuclei exchanging the energy given to them by the RF pulse to their surrounding environment. The efficiency of this process determines the T1 time of the tissue in which they are situated.
• Owing to the fact that fat is able to absorb energy quickly (*see* Chapter 5), **the T1 time of fat is very short**, i.e. nuclei dispose of their energy to the surrounding fat tissue and return to B_0 in a short time.

T1 recovery in water
• Water is very inefficient at receiving energy from nuclei (*see* Chapter 5). **The T1 time of water is therefore quite long**, i.e. nuclei take a lot longer to dispose of their energy to the surrounding water tissue and return to B_0.
• The TR controls how much of the NMV in fat or water has recovered before the application of the next RF pulse (Fig. 6.2).

Short TRs do not permit full longitudinal recovery in either fat or water so that there are different longitudinal components in fat and water.

These different longitudinal components are converted to different transverse components after the next excitation pulse has been applied. As the NMV does not recover completely to the positive longitudinal

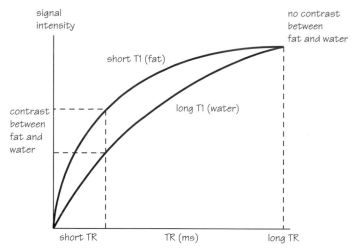

Fig. 6.2 The T1 differences between fat and water.

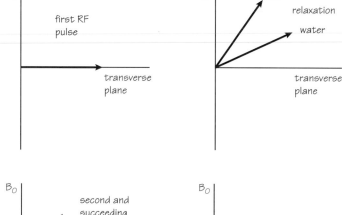

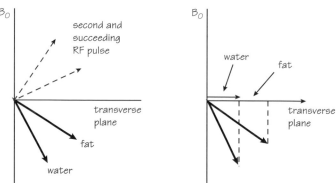

Fig. 6.3 Saturation.

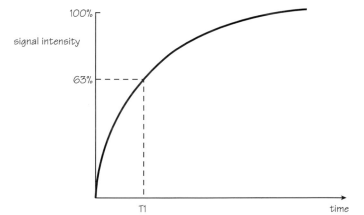

Fig. 6.1 The T1 recovery curve.

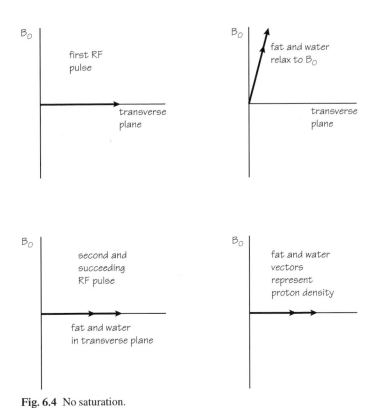

Fig. 6.4 No saturation.

axis, they are pushed beyond the transverse plane by the succeeding 90° RF pulse. This is called **saturation** (Fig. 6.3). When saturation occurs there is a contrast difference between fat and water due to differences in T1 recovery using short TRs.

Long TRs allow full recovery of the longitudinal components in fat and water. There is no difference in the magnitude of their longitudinal components. There is no contrast difference between fat and water due to differences in T1 recovery when using long TRs. Any differences seen in contrast are due to differences in the number of protons or **proton density** of each tissue (Fig. 6.4). The proton density of a particular tissue is an intrinsic contrast parameter and is therefore inherent to the tissue being imaged.

7 T2 decay

T2 decay is caused by the exchange of energy from one nucleus to another. It is called **spin–spin energy transfer**. It occurs as a result of the intrinsic magnetic fields of the nuclei interacting with each other. This energy exchange produces a loss of phase coherence or dephasing, and results in decay of the NMV in the transverse plane. It is an exponential process and occurs at different rates in different tissues.

The **T2 decay time** of a particular tissue is an intrinsic contrast parameter and is inherent to the tissue being imaged. It is the time it takes for 63% of the transverse magnetization to be lost due to dephasing, i.e. transverse magnetization is reduced to 63% of its original value (37% remains) (Fig. 7.1). The period of time over which this occurs is the time between the excitation pulse and the MR signal or the **TE**. The TE therefore determines how much T2 decay occurs in a particular tissue.

T2 decay in fat and water

T2 relaxation occurs as a result of the spins of adjacent nuclei interacting with each other and exchanging energy. The efficiency of this process depends on how closely the molecular motion of the atoms matches the Larmor frequency and the proximity of other spins.

• The Larmor frequency is relatively low and therefore fat is much better at this energy exchange than water, whose molecular motion is much faster than the Larmor frequency and whose atoms are closely spaced (*see* Chapter 5). **Fat's T2 time is therefore very short compared with that of water**.
• The TE controls how much transverse magnetization has been allowed to decay in fat and water when the signal is read.

Short TEs do not permit full dephasing in either fat or water so their transverse components are similar. There is little contrast difference between fat and water due to differences in T2 decay using short TEs.

Long TEs allow dephasing of the transverse components in fat and water. There is a contrast difference between fat and water due to differences in T2 decay times when using long TEs.

It should be noted that fat and water represent the extremes in image contrast. Other tissues, such as muscle, grey matter and white matter have contrast characteristics that fall between fat and water (Fig. 7.2).

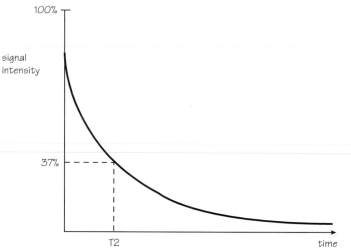

Fig. 7.1 The T2 decay curve.

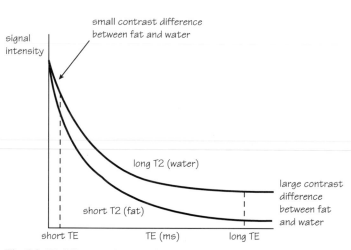

Fig. 7.2 T2 differences between fat and water.

8 T1 weighting

All three intrinsic contrast mechanisms affect image contrast, regardless of the pulse sequence, TR and TE used. For example, tissues with a low proton density, such as air, are always dark on an MR image and tissues in which nuclei move may be dark or bright depending on their velocity and the pulse sequence used. In order to produce images where the contrast is predictable, parameters are selected to **weight** the image towards one contrast mechanism and away from the other two.

T1 weighting

In a **T1 weighted image**, differences in the T1 relaxation times of tissues must be demonstrated. To achieve this a TR is selected that is short enough to ensure that the NMV in neither fat nor water has had time to relax back to B_0 before the application of the next excitation pulse. If the TR is long, the NMV in both fat and water recovers and their respective T1 relaxation times can no longer be distinguished.

• A **T1 weighted image** is an image whose contrast is predominantly due to the differences in T1 recovery times of tissues.

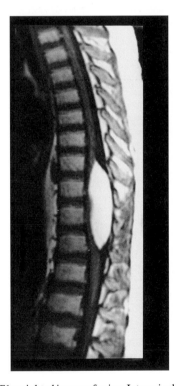

Fig. 8.1 Sagittal T1 weighted image of spine. Intraspinal lipoma is bright as it contains fat.

• For **T1 weighting** differences between the T1 times of tissues is exaggerated and to achieve this the **TR** must be **short**. To diminish T2 effects the TE must also be **short** (Fig. 8.1).

• In T1 weighted images, tissues with short T1 relaxation times such as **fat**, are **bright** (high signal), because they recover most of their longitudinal magnetization during the TR and therefore more magnetization is available to be flipped into the transverse plane by the next RF pulse.

• Tissues with long T1 relaxation times such as **water**, are **dark** (low signal) because they do not recover much of their longitudinal magnetization during the TR and therefore less magnetization is available to be flipped into the transverse plane by the next RF pulse.

• T1 weighted images best demonstrate anatomy but also show pathology if used after contrast enhancement.

Typical parameters
TR 300–600 ms (shorter in gradient echo sequences)
TE 10–30 ms (shorter in gradient echo sequences)

Table 8.1 Signal intensities seen in T1 weighted images.

High signal	fat
	haemangioma
	intra-osseous lipoma
	radiation change
	degeneration fatty deposition
	methaemoglobin
	cysts with proteinaceous fluid
	paramagnetic contrast agents
	slow flowing blood
Low signal	cortical bone
	avascular necrosis
	infarction
	infection
	tumours
	sclerosis
	cysts
	calcification
No signal	air
	fast flowing blood
	tendons
	cortical bone
	scar tissue
	calcification

9 T2 weighting

All three intrinsic contrast parameters affect image contrast regardless of the pulse sequence, TR and TE used. For example, tissues with a low proton density such as air, are always dark on an MR image and tissues in which nuclei move may be dark or bright depending on their velocity and the pulse sequence used. Therefore parameters are selected to **weight** the image towards one contrast mechanism and away from the other two.

T2 weighting

In a **T2 weighted image** the differences in the T2 relaxation times of tissues must be demonstrated. To achieve this, a TE is selected that is long enough to ensure that the NMV in both fat and water have had time to decay. If the TE is too short, the NMV in neither fat nor water has had time to decay and their respective T2 times cannot be distinguished.

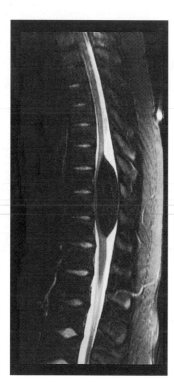

Fig. 9.1 Sagittal T2 weighted image through the spine in the same patient seen in Fig. 8.1. The intraspinal lipoma is now dark.

- A **T2 weighted image** is an image whose contrast is predominantly due to the differences in the T2 decay times of tissues.
- For **T2 weighting** the differences between the T2 times of tissues is exaggerated, therefore the **TE** must be **long**. T1 effects are diminished by selecting **a long TR** (Fig. 9.1).
- Tissues with a short T2 decay time such as **fat** are **dark** (low signal) because they lose most of their coherent transverse magnetization during the TE period.
- Tissues with a long T2 decay time such as **water** are **bright** (high signal), because they retain most of their transverse coherence during the TE period.
- T2 weighted images best demonstrate pathology as most pathology has an increased water content and is therefore bright on T2 weighted images.

Typical parameters
TR 2000 ms +
TE 70 ms +

Table 9.1 Signal intensities seen in T2 weighted images.

High signal	CSF
	synovial fluid
	haemangioma
	infection
	inflammation
	oedema
	some tumours
	haemorrhage
	slow-flowing blood
	cysts
Low signal	cortical bone
	bone islands
	de-oxyhaemoglobin
	haemosiderin
	calcification
	T2 paramagnetic agents
No signal	air
	fast flowing blood
	tendons
	cortical bone
	scar tissue
	calcification

10 Proton density weighting

All three intrinsic contrast parameters affect image contrast regardless of the pulse sequence, TR and TE used. Therefore parameters are selected to **weight** the image towards one contrast mechanism and away from the other two.

Proton density (PD) weighting

In a **PD weighted image** differences in the proton densities (number of hydrogen protons in the tissue) must be demonstrated. To achieve this both T1 and T2 effects are diminished. T1 effects are reduced by selecting a long TR and T2 effects are diminished by selecting a short TE.

• A **proton density weighted image** is an image whose contrast is predominantly due to differences in the proton density of the tissues (Fig. 10.1).

• Tissues with a **low proton density** are **dark** (low signal) because the low number of protons result in a small component of transverse magnetization.

• Tissues with a **high proton density** are **bright** (high signal) because the high number of protons result in a large component of transverse magnetization.

• Cortical bone and air are always dark on MR images regardless of the weighting as they have a low proton density and therefore return little signal.

• Proton density weighted images show anatomy and some pathology (Fig. 10.2).

Typical values
TR 2000 ms+
TE 10–30 ms

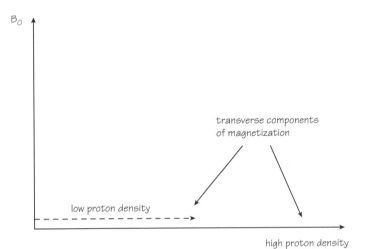

Fig. 10.1 Proton density contrast.

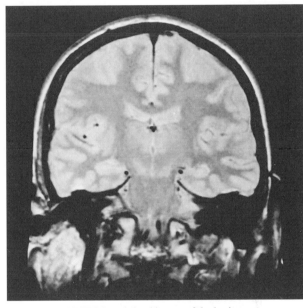

Fig. 10.2 Coronal FSE PD weighted image of the brain.

11 Pulse sequence mechanisms

A **pulse sequence** is defined as a series of RF pulses, gradients applications and intervening time periods. They enable control of the way in which the system applies RF pulses and gradients. By selecting the intervening time periods, image weighting is controlled (see Chapter 5). Pulse sequences are required because without a mechanism of refocusing spins, there is insufficient signal to produce an image. This is because dephasing occurs almost immediately after the RF excitation pulse has been removed.

Spins lose their phase coherence in two ways:
• by the interactions of the intrinsic magnetic fields of adjacent nuclei; **spin–spin energy transfer** (see Chapter 5);
• by the **inhomogeneities** of the external magnetic field.

Despite attempts to make the main magnetic field as uniform as possible via shimming (see Chapter 43), inhomogeneities of the external magnetic field are inevitable and slightly alter the magnitude of B_0, i.e. some small areas of the field have a magnetic field strength of slightly more or less than the main field strength (Fig. 11.1).

Owing to the Larmor equation, spins that pass through inhomogeneities experience a precessional frequency and phase change and the resulting signal decays exponentially. It is called a FID and its rate of decay is termed **T2*** (Fig. 11.2). Magnetic field inhomogeneities cause the NMV to dephase before intrinsic magnetic fields of the nuclei can produce dephasing, i.e. T2* happens before T2.

The main purposes of pulse sequences are:
• to rephase spins and remove inhomogeneity effects and therefore produce a signal or echo that contains information on the decay characteristics of tissue;
• to enable manipulation of the TE and TR to produce different types of contrast.

Spins are rephased in two ways (Tables 11.1 and 11.2):
• by using a 180° RF pulse
• by using a gradient.

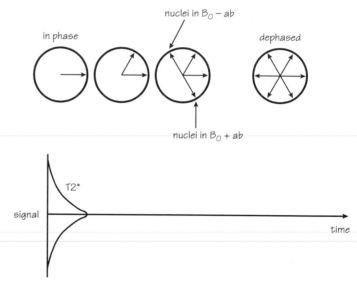

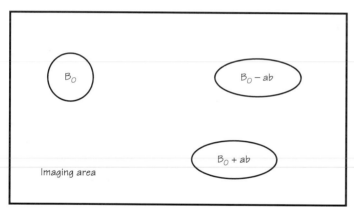

Fig. 11.1 Magnetic field inhomogeneities (ab represents these areas).

Fig. 11.2 T2* decay.

Table 11.1 Pulse sequences and their rephasing mechanisms.

Use 180° pulses to rephase spins	Use gradients to rephase spins
Spin echo	gradient echo
Fast spin echo	coherent gradient echo
Inversion recovery	incoherent gradient echo
STIR	steady state free precession
FLAIR	ultrafast sequences

Table 11.2 Comparison of gradient echo and spin echo sequences.

Spin echo	Gradient echo
Uses a RF pulse to rephase	uses a gradient to rephase
Uses flip angles of 90°	uses variable flip angles
Inhomogeneity effects are eliminated	inhomogeneity effects are not eliminated
Is a slow sequence	is a fast sequence

12 The conventional spin echo pulse sequence (SE)

Conventional spin echo pulse sequences are used to produce T1, T2 or proton density weighted images and are one of the most basic pulse sequences used in MRI. In a spin echo pulse sequence there is a 90° excitation pulse followed by a 180° rephasing pulse followed by an **echo** (Fig. 12.1)

Mechanisms

• After the application of the 90° RF pulse, spins lose precessional coherence because of an increase or decrease in their precessional frequency caused by the magnetic field inhomogeneities. The NMV decays in the transverse plane and the ability to generate a signal is lost.
• Spins that experience an increase in precessional frequency gain phase relative to those that experience a decrease in precessional frequency which lag behind. Dephasing can be imagined as a 'fan' where spins that lag behind are slow, whereas those that gain phase are fast.
• A 180° RF pulse flips the dephased nuclei through 180°. The fast edge is now behind the slow edge. The fast edge eventually catches up with the slow edge reforming the NMV. This is called **rephasing**.

• The signal in the receiver coil is regenerated and can be measured. This regenerated signal is called an echo and, because an RF pulse has been used to generate it, it is specifically called a **spin echo**.
• Rephasing the NMV eliminates the effect of the magnetic field inhomogeneities. Whenever a 180° RF rephasing pulse is applied, a spin echo results. Rephasing pulses may be applied either once or several times to produce either one or several spin echoes.

Contrast

CSE are usually used in one of two ways as follows.

A **single spin echo** pulse consists of a single 180° RF pulse applied after the excitation pulse to produce a single spin echo. This a typical sequence used to produce a T1 weighted set of images (Fig. 12.2).
• The **TR** is the length of time from one 90° RF pulse to the next 90° RF pulse. For T1 weighted imaging a short TR is used.
• The **TE** is the length of time from the 90° RF pulse that begins the pattern to the mid-point or peak of the signal generated after the 180° RF pulse, i.e. the spin echo. For T1 weighted imaging a short TE is used.

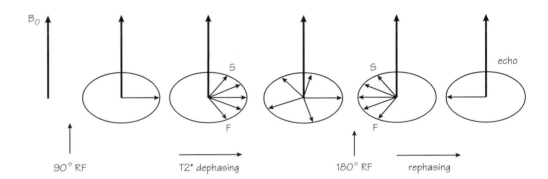

Fig. 12.1 RF rephasing.

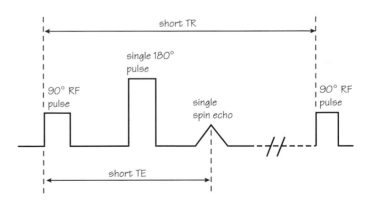

Fig. 12.2 What weighting do you think this spin echo will have?

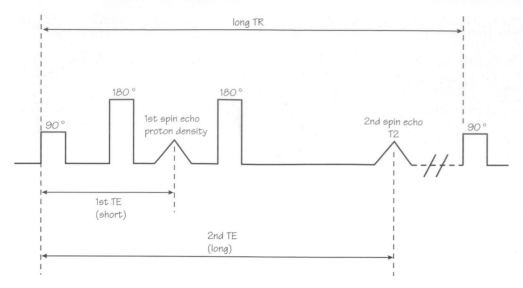

Fig. 12.3 A dual echo pulse sequence.

A **dual echo sequence** consists of two 180° pulses applied to produce two spin echoes (Fig. 12.3). This is a sequence that provides two images per slice location; one that is proton density weighted and one that is T2 weighted.

• The first echo has a short TE (TE1) and a long TR and results in a set of proton density weighted images.

• The second echo has a long TE (TE2) and a long TR and results in a T2 weighted set of images. This echo has less amplitude than the first echo because more T2 decay has occurred by this point.

Typical parameters

Single echo (for T1 weighting)

TR	300–500 ms
TE	10–30 ms (Fig. 12.4)

Dual echo (for PD/T2 weighting)

TR	2000+ ms
TE1	20 ms
TE2	80 ms (Fig. 12.5)

Uses

Spin echo sequences are still considered the gold standard in that the contrast they produce is understood and is predictable. They produce T1, T2 and PD weighted images of good quality and may be used in any part of the body for any indication.

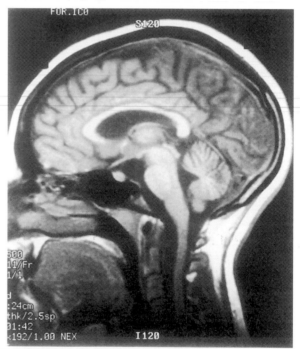

Fig. 12.4 T1 weighted sagittal image of the brain, TE 11 ms, TR 500 ms.

Advantages	Disadvantages
Good image quality	Long scan times
Very versatile	
True T2 weighting	
Available on all systems	
Gold standard for image contrast and weighting	

Fig. 12.5 (a) A proton density weighted axial image of the brain, TE 20 ms, TR 2700 ms. (b) A T2 weighted coronal image of the brain, TE 90 ms, TR 2700 ms.

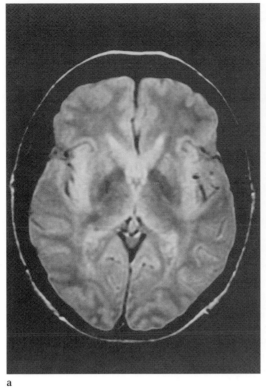

a

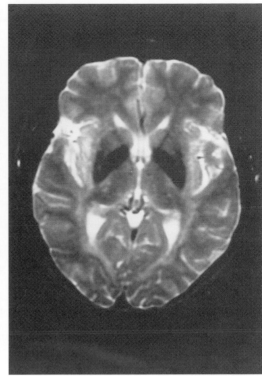

b

13 Fast or turbo spin echo (FSE/TSE)

Fast spin echo (FSE) is a much faster version of conventional spin echo. In spin echo sequences, one phase encoding only is performed during each TR (see Chapter 23). The scan time is a function of TR, NEX and phase encodings. One of the ways of speeding up a conventional sequence is to reduce the number of phase encoding steps. However this normally results in a loss of resolution. FSE overcomes this by still performing the same number of phase encodings, thereby maintaining resolution, but more than one phase encoding is performed per TR, reducing the scan time.

Mechanism

• FSE employs a train of 180° rephasing pulses, each one producing a spin echo. This train of spin echoes is called an **echo train**. The number of 180° RF pulses and resultant echoes is called the **echo train length (ETL)** or **turbo factor**. The spacing between each echo is called the **echo spacing**.

• After each rephasing, a phase encoding step is performed and data from the resultant echo are stored in K space (see Chapters 26 and 27) (Fig. 13.1). Therefore several lines of K space are filled every TR instead of one line as in conventional spin echo. As K space is filled more rapidly, the scan time decreases.

• Typically 2, 4, 8 or 16, 180° RF pulses are applied during every TR. As 2, 4, 8 or 16 phase encodings are also performed during each TR, the scan time is reduced to 1/2, 1/4, 1/8 or 1/16 of the original scan time. The **higher** the turbo factor the **shorter** the scan time (Table 13.1).

Contrast

• Each echo has a different TE and data from each echo are used to produce one image (as opposed to dual echo CSE when two echoes have different TEs but produce two sets of images, one PD and the other T2). There would normally be a mixture of contrast.

• In any sequence, each phase encoding step applies a different slope of phase gradient to phase shift each slice by a different amount. This ensures data are placed in a different line of K space.

• The very **steep** gradient slopes significantly **reduce the amplitude** of the resultant echo/signal because they reduce the rephasing effect of the 180° rephasing pulse. **Shallow** gradients on the other hand do not have this effect and the amplitude of the resultant **echo/signal is at a maximum** (Fig. 13.2).

• When the TE is selected (known as the **effective TE** in FSE sequences) the resultant image must have a weighting corresponding to that TE, i.e. if the TE is set at 102 ms a T2 weighted image is obtained (assuming the TR is long).

• The system therefore orders the phase encodings (Fig. 13.3) so that those that produce the most signal (the shallowest ones) are used on echoes produced from 180° pulses nearest to the effective TE selected. The steepest gradients (which reduce the signal) are reserved for those echoes that are produced by 180° pulses furthest away from the effective TE. Therefore the resultant image is mostly made from data acquired at approximately the correct TE, although some other data are present.

Owing to different contrasts being present in the image, the contrast of FSE is unique.

• In T2 weighted scans, water and fat are hyperintense (bright). This is because the succession of 180° RF pulses reduces the spin–spin interactions in fat thereby increasing its T2 decay time (**J coupling**).

Table 13.1 FSE time saving illustrations.

Pulse sequence	Scan time
CSE, 256 phase encodings, 1NEX	$256 \times 1 \times TR$ $= 256 \times TR$
FSE, 256 phase encodings, 1 NEX and ETL 16	$256 \times 1 \times TR/16$ $= 16 \times TR$

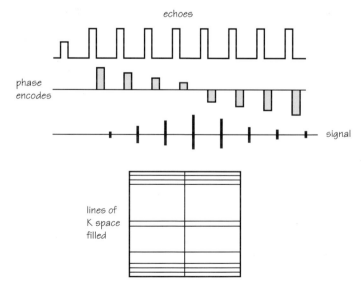

Fig. 13.1 K space filling in fast spin echo.

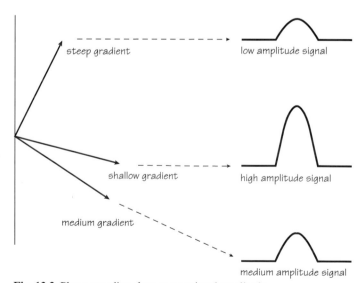

Fig. 13.2 Phase encoding slope versus signal amplitude.

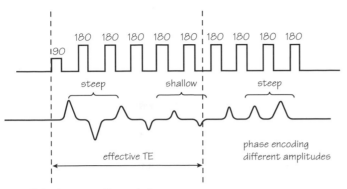

Fig. 13.3 Phase encoding ordering.

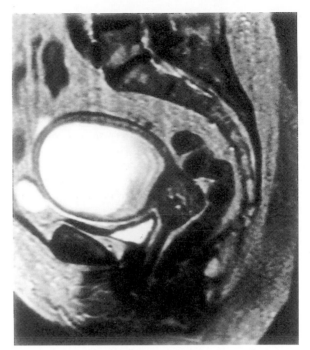

Fig. 13.5 Sagittal T2 weighted fast spin echo sequence of the pelvis, TE 102 ms, TR 4000 ms, turbo factor 16. Scan time 2 min 8 s.

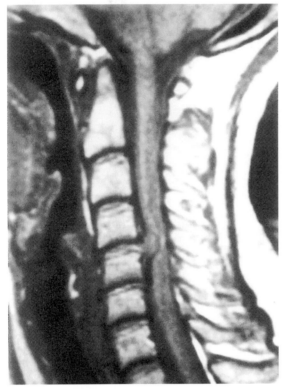

Fig. 13.4 Sagittal T1 weighted fast spin echo sequence of the cervical spine, TE 17 ms, TR 500 ms, turbo factor 4. Scan time 2 min 36 s.

Techniques used to suppress fat signal are therefore sometimes required to differentiate fat and pathology in T2 weighted FSE sequences.

• Muscle is often darker than in conventional spin echo T2 weighted images. This is because the succession of RF pulses increases **magnetization transfer** effects that produce saturation.

• In T1 weighted imaging, CNR is sometimes reduced so that the images look rather 'flat'. It is therefore best used when inherent contrast is good.

Typical parameters

Dual echo
TR 2500–4500 ms (for weighting and slice number)
effective TE1 17 ms
effective TE2 102 ms
ETL 8 – This may be split so that the PD image is acquired with the first four echoes and the T2 with the second four.

Single echo T2 weighting
TR 4000–8000 ms
TE 102 ms
ETL 16

Single echo T1 weighting
TR 600 ms
TE 17 ms
ETL 4

Uses

FSE produces T1, T2 or proton density scans in a fraction of the time of CSE. Because the scan times are reduced, matrix size can be increased to improve spatial resolution. FSE is usually used for brains, spines (Fig. 13.4), joints, extremities and the pelvis (Fig. 13.5). As FSE is incompatible with respiratory compensation techniques, it can only be used in the chest and abdomen with respiratory triggering or multiple NEX.

Systems that have sufficiently powerful gradients can use FSE in a single shot mode (see Chapter 27), or via slightly slower version called multi-shot. Both of these techniques permit image acquisition in a single breath-hold. In addition using very long TEs and TRs permit very heavy T2 weighting (**watergrams**).

Advantages	Disadvantages
Short scan times	Some flow artefacts increased
High resolution imaging	Incompatible with some imaging options
Increased T2 weighting	Some contrast interpretation problems
Magnetic susceptibility decreases*	Image blurring possible

* This can be a disadvantage as well as an advantage, e.g. haemorrhage.

14 Inversion recovery (IR)

Inversion recovery sequences were initially designed to produce very heavy T1 weighting. However at present they are mainly used in conjunction with a FSE sequence to produce T2 weighted images. Both are described here.

Mechanism

• Inversion recovery is a spin echo sequence that begins with a 180° inverting pulse (Fig. 14.1). This inverts the NMV through 180°. The TR is the time between successive 180° inverting pulses.
• When the pulse is removed the NMV begins to relax back to B_0. A 90° pulse is then applied at time interval **TI (time from inversion)** after the 180° inverting pulse.
• A further 180° RF pulse is applied which rephases spins in the transverse plane and produces an echo at time TE after the excitation pulse.

Contrast

• The TI is the main factor that controls weighting in IR sequences. If the TI is sufficiently long to allow the NMV to pass through the transverse plane, the contrast depends on the degree of saturation that is produced by the 90° pulse (as in spin echo), i.e. if the 90° pulse is applied shortly after the NMV has passed through the transverse plane, heavy saturation and T1 weighting results. TIs of 300 ms to 700 ms result in this type of heavy T1 weighting (Fig. 14.2). Certain TI values result in suppression of signal from tissues.
• The TE controls the amount of T2 decay. For T1 weighting it must be short, for T2 weighting, long.
• The TR must always be long enough to allow full longitudinal recovery of magnetization before each inverting pulse.

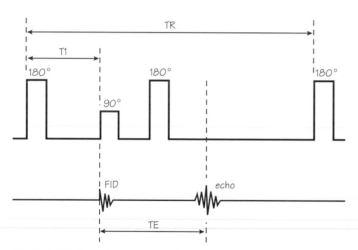

Fig. 14.1 The inversion recovery pulse sequence.

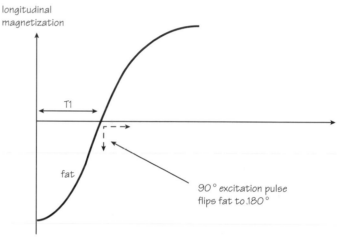

Fig. 14.3 STIR.

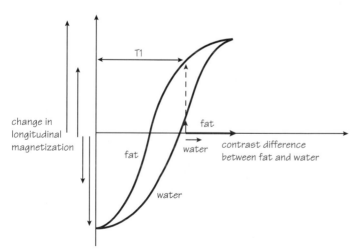

Fig. 14.2 T1 weighting in inversion recovery.

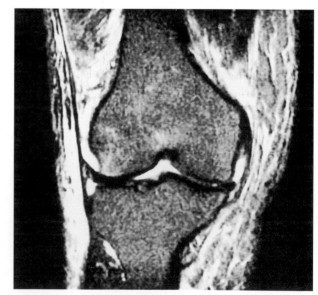

Fig. 14.4 Coronal STIR image of the knee. Note the high signal intensity in the soft tissues around the joint.

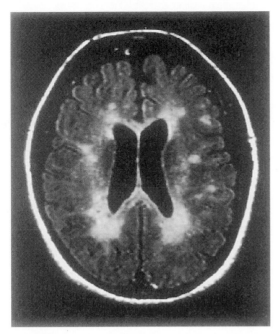

Fig. 14.5 A T2 weighted fast FLAIR image of the brain using TE 140 ms, TR 4600 ms and TI 1750 ms. The long TI has suppressed the signal from CSF improving the visualisation of the peri-ventricular MS plaques.

Fast inversion recovery is a combination of inversion recovery and fast spin echo. In this sequence the NMV is flipped through 180° into full saturation by a 180° inverting pulse. As in conventional inversion recovery, the TR is the time between each successive 180° pulse. At a time T1, the 90° excitation pulse is applied. However, after this, multiple 180° rephasing pulses are applied to produce multiple echoes which are phase encoded with a different slope of gradient. As in fast spin echo, multiple lines of K space are filled each TR, thereby significantly reducing the scan time. This modification of inversion recovery is now used in preference to the conventional sequence because, as the TR required for IR sequences must be increased in order to permit full recovery of the longitudinal magnetization, scan times are very long. Fast IR allows much shorter scan times to be implemented. The parameters used are similar to conventional IR except that the ETL or turbo factor must be selected. This should be short for T1 weighting and long for T2 weighting.

With both sequence types a further modification of the TI allows suppression of signal from various tissue types.

STIR (short TI inversion recovery) uses short TIs such as 100–180 ms, depending on field strength (Fig. 14.3). TIs of this magnitude place the 90° excitation pulse at the time that NMV of fat is passing exactly through the transverse plane. At this point (called the **null point**) there is no longitudinal component in fat. Therefore the 90° excitation pulse produces no transverse component in fat and therefore no signal. In this way a fat suppressed image results (Fig. 14.4).

FLAIR (fluid attenuated inversion recovery) uses long TIs such as 1700–2200 ms, depending on field strength, to null the signal from CSF in exactly the same way as the STIR sequence (Fig. 14.5). Because CSF has a long T1 recovery time, the TI must be longer to correspond with its null point.

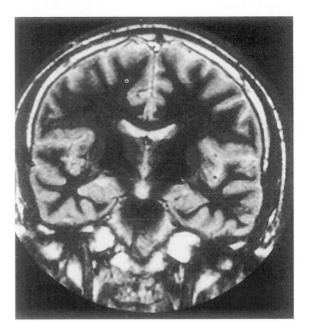

Fig. 14.6 A coronal T1 weighted inversion recovery sequence, TI 400 ms, TE 10 ms, TR 2000 ms.

Typical parameters

The required TI depends on the field strength (higher at higher fields).

T1 weighting (Fig. 14.6)
TI 300–700 ms
TE 10–20 ms
TR long
ETL 4

STIR (Fig. 14.4)
TI 100–180 ms
TE 70 ms+ (for T2 weighting)
TR long
ETL 16

FLAIR (Fig. 14.5)
TI 1500–2200 ms
TE 70 ms+ (for T2 weighting)
TR long
ETL 12–16

Uses

Inversion recovery is a very versatile sequence that is mainly used in the CNS (T1 and FLAIR) and musculoskeletal systems (STIR). The FLAIR sequence increases the conspicuity of periventricular lesions such as MS plaques and lesions in the cervical and thoracic cord. STIR sequences are often called 'search and destroy' sequences when used in the musculoskeletal system as they null the signal from normal marrow thereby increasing the conspicuity of bone lesions.

Advantages	Disadvantages
Versatile	Long scan times (conventional SE)
Good image quality	
Sensitive to pathology	

15 Gradient echo mechanisms

Gradient echo pulse sequences are sequences that use a gradient to reduce magnetic homogeneity effects, as opposed to a 180° RF pulse used in spin echo sequences.

Mechanism

• The radio frequency excitation and relaxation pattern used in gradient echo consists of an RF excitation pulse followed by a relaxation period and a gradient reversal to produce rephasing of the spins. The magnitude and duration of the RF excitation pulse selected determines the **flip angle**, i.e. the angle through which the NMV moves away from B_0 during resonance (Fig. 15.1).

• A transverse component of magnetization is created, the magnitude of which is less than in spin echo, where all the longitudinal magnetization is converted to the transverse plane. When a flip angle other than

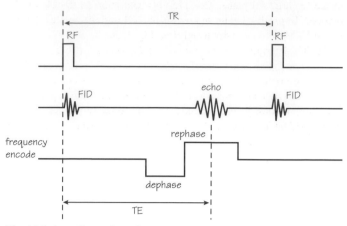

Fig. 15.3 A gradient echo pulse sequence.

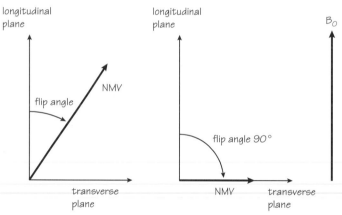

Fig. 15.1 The flip angle. What flip angle will give the maximum transverse magnetization?

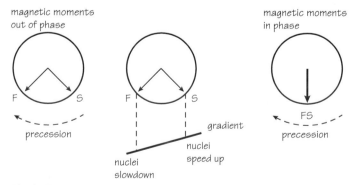

Fig. 15.2 How gradients rephase.

90° is used, only part of the longitudinal magnetization is converted to transverse magnetization, which precesses in the transverse plane and induces a signal in the receiver coil. Therefore the SNR in gradient echo sequences is less than in spin echo sequences.

• After the RF pulse is withdrawn, the FID is immediately produced as a result of inhomogeneities in the magnetic field. T2* dephasing therefore occurs before T1 and T2 processes have had time to develop.

• The magnetic moments within the transverse component of magnetization dephase and are then rephased by a **gradient** (Fig. 15.2).

• A gradient causes a change in the magnetic field strength that changes the precessional frequency and phase of spins. This effect rephases the magnetic moments so that a signal is received by the coil that contains T1 and T2 information. This signal is called a **gradient echo**.

• Gradient rephasing is less efficient than RF rephasing. Gradient rephasing does not reverse all of the dephased nuclei. Some nuclei that have been dephased from T2* are not rephased. Gradient echo images therefore contain some residual T2* effects. However, gradient rephasing is faster than RF rephasing and therefore these sequences have shorter TEs and TRs than spin echo. As a result scan times are short.

In a gradient echo pulse sequence (Fig. 15.3), rephasing is performed by the **frequency encoding gradient** (Chapter 24).

• The nuclei are dephased with a negative gradient pulse. The negative gradient slows down the slow nuclei even further and speeds up the fast ones. This accelerates the dephasing process.

• The gradient polarity is then reversed to positive. The positive gradient speeds up the slow nuclei and slows down the fast ones. The nuclei rephase and produce a gradient echo.

• Gradient echo images are more sensitive to external magnetic field imperfections because T2* dephasing effects, produced by these inhomogeneities, are not totally eliminated by gradient rephasing.

Contrast

As in spin echo imaging, the TR controls T1 weighting. The TR used in gradient echo is usually much shorter than in spin echo. This normally increases saturation and therefore T1 weighting. To overcome this, the flip angle is reduced to less than 90° so that the NMV is predominantly in the longitudinal plane. This prevents saturation so the TR can be reduced. **In gradient echo sequences the TR and flip angle together control T1/proton density weighting** (Fig. 15.4).

The TE determines the amount of T2 dephasing that occurs before the NMV is rephased and therefore the amount of T2 relaxation affecting image contrast. The longer the TE, the more T2 contrast in the image. As gradient rephasing is less efficient than RF rephasing at removing inhomogeneity effects, gradient echo sequences contain more residual T2* effects than spin echo. As a result the term T2* weighting is used in gradient echo imaging. **In gradient echo sequences the TE controls T2* weighting.**

Typical parameters
(Table 15.1)
T1 weighting (Fig. 15.5)
• Use a TR and flip angle to produce maximum T1 effects. The flip angle must shift the majority of the NMV towards the transverse plane to produce saturation. **The flip angle must be large.**
• The TR must not permit nuclei in the majority of tissues to recover to the longitudinal axis prior to the repetition of the next RF excitation pulse. Therefore the **TR must be short**.
• Use a TE to produce minimum T2* effects. The TE should limit the amount of dephasing that occurs before the echo is regenerated. Therefore the **TE must be short**.

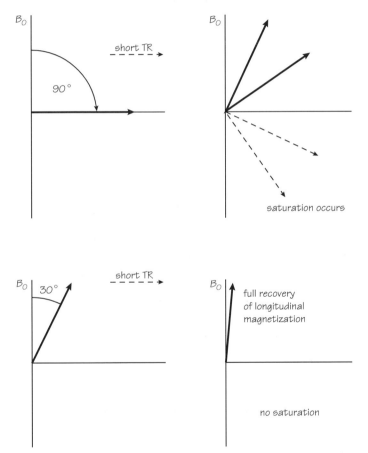

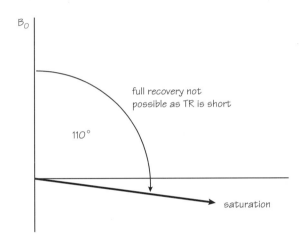

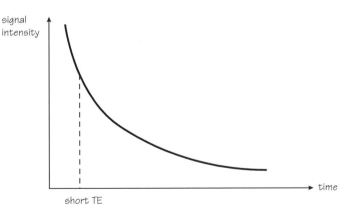

Fig. 15.4 How the TR and the flip angle control weighting.

Fig. 15.5 T1 weighting in gradient echo.

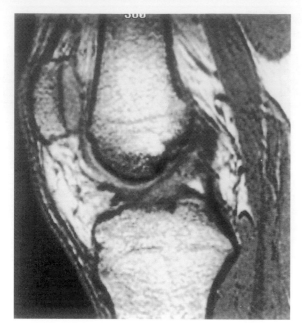

Fig. 15.6 A sagittal T1/proton density weighted image of the knee.

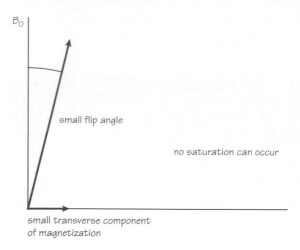

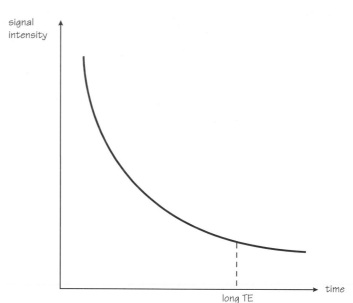

Fig. 15.7 T2* weighting in gradient echo.

For T1 weighting
TR less than 50 ms (short)
Flip angle 60–120° (large)
TE 5–10 ms (short) (Fig. 15.6)

T2* weighting (Fig. 15.7)
• The TE should permit maximum dephasing to occur before the signal is generated to produce maximum T2* effects. **The TE must be long.**
• The flip angle must shift only a minimum of the NMV towards the transverse plane. Small flip angles ensure that the majority of the net magnetization components remain in the longitudinal axis to prevent saturation. **The flip angle must be small**.
• **The TR must be long** enough to prevent saturation but can be reduced without producing significant saturation because of the small flip angle.

For T2* weighting
TR less than 500 ms (long)
Flip angle less than 30° (small)
TE 15–20 ms (relatively long) (Fig. 15.8)

Proton density weighting
• Select TR and flip angle to produce minimum T1 effects and a TE to produce minimum T2*/T2 effects. As a result proton density predominates. The **flip angle must be small** so that the majority of the NMV remains in the longitudinal axis and therefore saturation and T1 weighting is minimized.
• **The TR must be long** to minimize saturation and T1 effects as well.
• **The TE must be short** to minimize the T2*/T2 effects.

For proton density weighting
TR 200–600 ms (long)
Flip angle 5–20° (small)
TE 5–15 ms (short)

The steady state

This is a situation when the TR is shorter than both the T1 and T2 relaxation times of all the tissues. Therefore there is no time for the transverse magnetization to decay before the pulse pattern is repeated again. The only process that has time to occur is T2*. Therefore the NMV does not move between repetition times. This is called **steady state** (Fig. 15.9). Because the transverse magnetization does not have time to decay, its magnitude accumulates over successive TRs. This **residual transverse magnetization** therefore affects image contrast. Tissues with long T2 times (mainly water) appear bright. Most gradient echo sequences utilize the steady state because the TRs are so short that the fastest scan times are achievable.

To maintain the steady state the TR must be between 22 ms and 50 ms and the flip angle between 30° and 45°.

Table 15.1 Parameters used in gradient echo.

	TR	TE	Flip angle
T1 weighting	short	short	large
T2 weighting	long	long	small
PD weighting	long	short	small

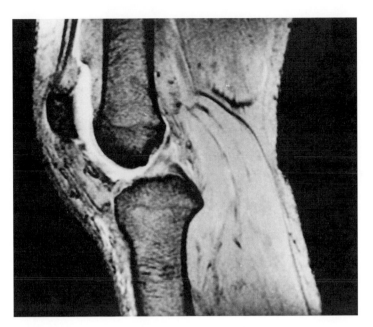

Fig. 15.8 Sagittal T2* weighted image of the knee showing normal appearances.

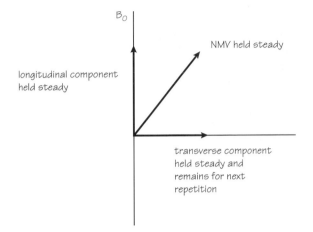

Fig. 15.9 The steady state.

16 Coherent gradient echo

Gradient echo pulse sequences can generally be categorized according to whether they utilize the steady state. The two main types of gradient echo sequence are called:
- **coherent** or rewind sequences;
- incoherent or spoiled sequences.

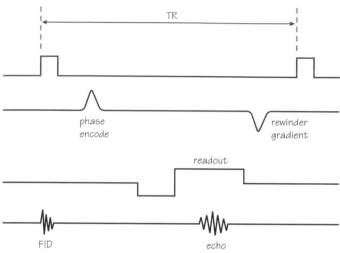

Fig. 16.1 The coherent gradient echo pulse sequence.

Mechanism

(Fig. 16.1)

This sequence uses:
- a gradient instead of a 180° rephasing pulse to regenerate the echo;
- the steady state by using very short TRs and medium flip angles so that there is residual transverse magnetization 'left over' when the next excitation pulse is delivered;
- a **rewinder/rephasing gradient** to amplify the effect of the residual magnetization. This gradient is a reversal of the phase encoding gradient. After the echo any residual transverse magnetization that still remains begins to dephase. The gradient used to phase encode at the beginning of the sequence is then switched on with opposite polarity and the same amplitude to the phase encode. This results in the residual transverse magnetization rephasing so that it is always in phase and therefore preserved when the next excitation pulse is applied. This process is called **rewinding** as it allows the residual transverse magnetization to build up and tissues with long T2 times are hyperintense on the image, e.g. blood, CSF, synovial fluid. These scans are often therefore said to produce an angiographic, myelographic or arthrographic appearance.

Typical parameters

As coherent gradient echo sequences utilize the steady state, the TR and the flip angle must be at values to achieve this. The TE determines how

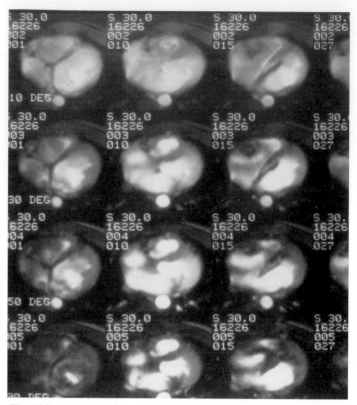

Fig. 16.2 Axial cine coherent GRE T2* weighted images of the heart.

much T2* has occurred when the echo is regenerated. Coherent gradient echo sequences are primarily used to achieve T2* weighting using the following parameters:

TR short (steady state)	40 ms
Flip angle medium (steady state)	30°
Long TE (maximize T2*)	20 ms

Uses

This sequence should be used when T2* weighted images (bright blood/water/CSF) are required with good temporal resolution (Fig. 16.2), as in:
- cine imaging of the heart;
- MRA; and
- volume imaging with T2 weighting.

Table 16.1 Coherent gradient echo acronyms.

Philips	FFE
GE	GRASS
Siemens	FISP

17 Incoherent sequences

Gradient echo pulse sequences can generally be categorized according to whether they utilize the steady state. The two main types of gradient echo sequence are called:
- coherent or rewind sequences; and
- **incoherent** or spoiled sequences.

Mechanism

This sequence:
- uses a gradient instead of a 180° rephasing pulse to regenerate the echo;
- utilizes the steady state by using very short TRs and medium flip angles so that there is residual transverse magnetization 'left over' when the next excitation pulse is delivered;
- eliminates this magnetization so that tissues with long T2 times are not allowed to dominate image contrast but T1/proton density contrast prevails; this is called **spoiling**;

Gradient spoiling involves applying a gradient that dephases the residual transverse magnetization (Fig. 17.1). **RF spoiling** applies RF excitation pulses at different phases every TR so that the residual transverse magnetization also has different phase values (and is therefore dephased).

Gradient spoiling is not as efficient as RF spoiling but T2* weighting can also be achieved. Gradient spoiled sequences are therefore more versatile than RF spoiled sequences.

Typical parameters

The incoherent gradient echo sequence utilizes the steady state, so the TR and the flip angle must be at values to achieve this. The TE is as short as possible to minimize T2* effects. Incoherent gradient echo is primarily used for T1 weighting with the following parameters:

TR short (steady state)	35 ms
Flip angle medium (steady state)	35°
Short TE (minimize T2*)	6 ms

Sometimes it is desirable to use gradient echo sequences out of the steady state using a TR comparable to spin echo. A gradient is still used to rephase the spins and variable flip angles are also utilized. However, selecting a TR of several hundred ms allows multiple slice acquisition with good SNR.

Uses

This sequence should be used when T1 weighted images are required with good temporal resolution (Fig. 17.2), as in:
- 3D volume acquisitions to acquire data from a volume of tissue. A whole slab is excited (but not slice selected) and during the encoding process the slab is phase shifted into slices (**slice encoding**). Volume acquisition allows very thin slices to be obtained at many slice locations. The data acquired can then be used to view the slab in any plane. 3D incoherent gradient echo is mainly used in the knee, brachial plexus and brain;
- 2D breathhold T1 weighted sequences; (Fig. 17.2)
- dynamic contrast enhanced images.

Table 17.1 Incoherent gradient echo acronyms.

Philips	T1 FFE
GE	SPGR
Siemens	FLASH

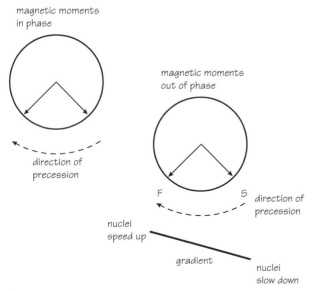

Fig. 17.1 How gradients dephase.

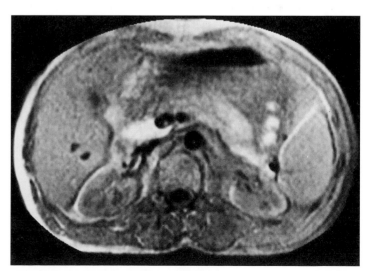

Fig. 17.2 Axial breath-hold T1 weighted incoherent (spoiled) GRE image showing normal appearances.

18 Steady state free precession (SSFP)

Gradient echo sequences do not demonstrate true T2 weighting because:
• the TE is never long enough;
• gradient rephasing is so inefficient, that any echo is dominated by T2* effects.

SSFP is a steady state sequence that obtains images that have a sufficiently long TE and less T2* when using the steady state than other gradient echo pulse sequences. This is achieved in the following manner.

Mechanism

• Any RF pulse contains radio-waves of differing amplitudes. The magnitude of the RF pulse is merely an average of these amplitudes so that a net effect is produced (Fig. 18.1). Every RF pulse, regardless of its net magnitude, contains a small number of radio-waves that, on their own, have sufficient magnitude to move magnetic moments within the NMV through 180°. These radio-waves are therefore able to rephase a FID.

• In SSFP, the steady state is maintained by using a flip angle between 30° and 45° in conjunction with a TR of less than 50 ms.

• Every TR an excitation pulse is applied. When the RF is switched off a FID is produced.

• After the TR, another excitation pulse is applied which also produces its own FID. However, the radio-waves within it that have an amplitude of 180° rephase the previous FID and a spin echo results (Fig. 18.2).

• Each RF pulse therefore not only produces its own FID, but also rephases the FID produced from the previous excitation.

As nuclei take as long to rephase as they took to dephase, the echo from the first excitation pulse occurs at the same time as the third excitation pulse. RF cannot be transmitted and received at the same time. To prevent this, a rewinder gradient is used to speed up the rephasing process after the RF rephasing has begun. Rewinding moves the echo (Fig. 18.3) so that it occurs before the next excitation pulse, rather than during it. In this way, the resultant echo can be received and data from it collected.

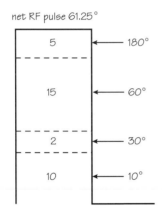

Fig. 18.1 The net effect of RF pulse energy.

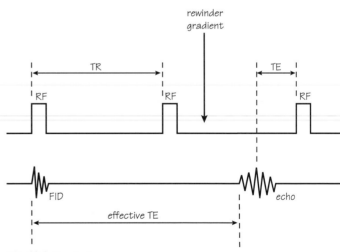

Fig. 18.3 Rewinding.

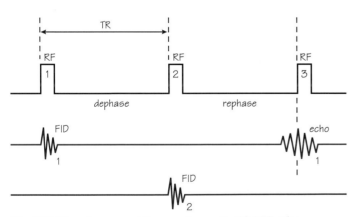

Fig. 18.2 The echo occurs at the same time as the third RF pulse.

The resultant echo demonstrates more true T2 weighting than conventional gradient echo sequences, for the following reasons.

• The TE is now longer than the TR. In SSFP, there are usually two TEs: the **actual TE** (time between the echo and the next excitation pulse) and the **effective TE** time from the echo to the excitation pulse that created its FID. Therefore the *effective TE* = $(2 \times TR)$ − actual TE and is long enough to measure the true T2. The actual TE affects the effective TE. The longer the actual TE, the lower the effective TE;

• Rephasing has been initiated by an RF pulse rather than a gradient so that more T2 and less T2* information is present. The rewinder gradient merely repositions the echo at a time when it can be received.

Typical values

Flip angle	30°–45°
TR	Less than 50 ms
Actual	TE 7 ms

Uses

SSFP sequences are used to acquire images that demonstrate true T2 weighting rapidly (Fig. 18.4). With the advent of fast spin echo, however, this sequence is not commonly used.

Table 18.1 Steady state free precession acronyms.

Philips	T2 FFE
GE	SSFP
Siemens	PSIF

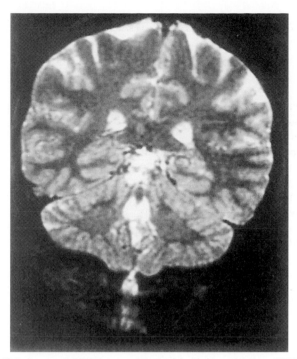

Fig. 18.4 A coronal SSFP image of the brain, effective TE 71 ms, TE 9 ms, TR 40 ms, flip angle 35°. This image was acquired as part of a volume acquisition and took 9 min to complete.

19 Ultrafast sequences

The most recent advances have been made in developing very fast pulse sequences that can acquire several slices in a single breath-hold. These usually employ much faster versions of coherent and incoherent gradient echo sequences or combinations of both (**hybrids**). Faster scan times are achieved in the following ways:
• applying only a portion of the RF excitation pulse, so that it takes much less time to apply and switch off;
• reading only a proportion of the echo (**partial echo**);
• using asymmetric gradients which are faster to apply than conventional balanced gradients;

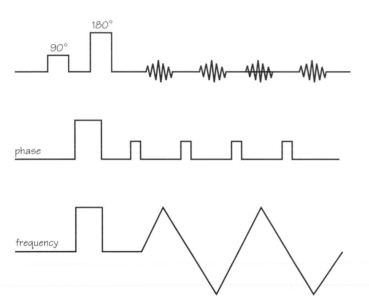

Fig. 19.1 Spin echo EPI.

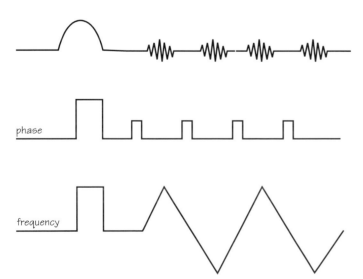

Fig. 19.2 Gradient echo EPI.

• sampling frequencies whilst the frequency encoding gradient is still rising (**ramped sampling**);
• filling K space in a single shot or in segments (see Chapter 27).

These measures ensure that the TE and TR are very short. TEs as low as 1 ms and TRs as low as 5 ms can be achieved in this manner enabling the whole abdomen to be imaged in a single breath-hold. In addition, many ultrafast sequences use extra pulses applied before the pulse sequence begins to pre-magnetize the tissue. In this way a certain contrast can be obtained. Pre-magnetization is usually achieved in two ways, as follows.
• A 180° pulse is applied before the pulse sequence begins. This inverts the NMV into full saturation and, at a specified delay time, the pulse sequence itself begins. This can be used to null signal from certain organs and tissues and is similar to inversion recovery. It is sometimes known as **a magnetization prepared** sequence.
• A 90°/180°/90° combination is applied before the pulse sequence begins. The first 90° pulse produces transverse magnetization. The 180° pulse rephases this, and at a specified time later the second 90° pulse is applied. This drives the coherent transverse magnetization into the longitudinal plane, so that it is available to be flipped when the pulse sequence begins. This is used to produce T2 contrast and is sometimes known as **driven equilibrium**.

Weighting is achieved in these sequences by applying all the shallowest phase encoding gradients first, and leaving the steep ones until the end of the pulse sequence. In this way, the effect of the pre-magnetization prevails as, when it is dominant, the central phase encodings (which produce the greatest signal amplitudes and determine the weighting of the sequence) are performed (see Chapter 25). By the end of the sequence, the pre-magnetization has decayed and this is when the low signal amplitudes are acquired.

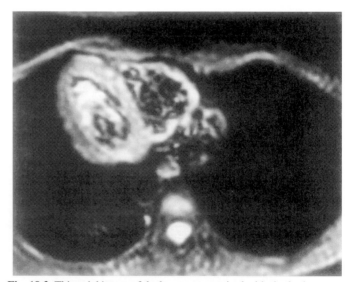

Fig. 19.3 This axial image of the heart was acquired with single shot EPI. Although the resolution of the image is marginal, this image was acquired in 20 ms.

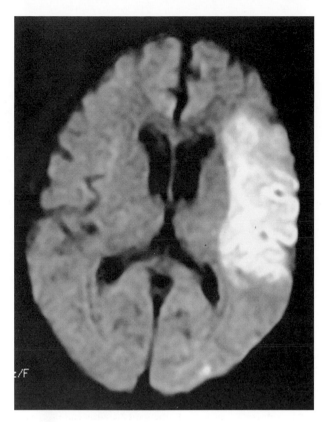

Fig. 19.4 Single shot EPI image of the brain. The entire brain was scanned in 14 s.

Echo planar imaging (EPI)

EPI is an MR acquisition method that collects all the data required to fill all the lines of K space from a single echo train. In order to achieve this, multiple echoes are generated and each is phase encoded by a different slope of gradient to fill all the required lines of K space. Echoes are generated either by 180° rephasing pulses (termed **spin echo EPI**) (Fig. 19.1), or by gradients (termed **gradient echo EPI**) (Fig. 19.2). Gradient rephasing is much faster and involves no RF deposition to the patient but does require high speed gradients. In order to fill all of K space in one repetition, the readout and phase encode gradients must rapidly switch on and off (see Chapter 27).

As data acquisition is so rapid in EPI, images may be acquired in 50 ms to 80 ms. Axial images of the whole brain are possible in 2 s to 3 s and whole body imaging in about 30 s. EPI sequences place exceptional strains on the gradients and therefore gradient modifications are required.

Typical parameters

Either proton density or T2 weighting is achieved by selecting either a short or long effective TE which corresponds to the time interval between the excitation pulse and when the centre of K space is filled. T1 weighting is possible by applying an inverting pulse prior to the excitation pulse to produce saturation.

Uses

Functional imaging
Real time cardiac imaging (Fig. 19.3)
Perfusion/diffusion (Fig. 19.4)

20 Specialist sequences

Diffusion weighted imaging

Diffusion is a term used to describe moving molecules due to random thermal motion. This motion is restricted by boundaries such as ligaments, membranes and macro-molecules (Fig. 20.1). In early stroke, cells swell and absorb water from the extra-cellular space and diffusion is restricted. **Diffusion weighted images** are acquired by combining EPI or fast gradient echo sequences with two large gradient pulses applied after excitation. The gradient pulses are designed to cancel each other out if spins do not move, whilst moving spins experience phase shift. Signal attenuation therefore occurs in normal tissues with random motion and high signal appears in tissues with restricted diffusion.

The amount of attenuation depends on the amplitude and the direction of the applied diffusion gradients. Diffusion gradients applied in the X, Y and Z axes are combined to produce a diffusion weighted image (isotropic image). When the diffusion gradients are applied in only one direction, signal changes reflect direction of axons (anisotropic image).

Diffusion gradients must be strong to achieve enough diffusion weighting. Diffusion sensitivity is controlled by a parameter 'b' that determines the diffusion attenuation by modification of the time duration and amplitude of the diffusion gradient. 'b' is expressed in units of s/mm^2. Typical 'b' values range from 500 s/mm^2 to 1000 s/mm^2.

Clinical applications

Diagnosis of stroke where areas of decreased diffusion, which represent infarction, are either dark or bright depending on the technique used (Fig. 20.2).

Perfusion imaging

Perfusion is a measure of the quality of vascular supply to a tissue. Since vascular supply and metabolism are usually related, perfusion can also be used to measure tissue activity. **Perfusion imaging** (Fig. 20.3) utilizes a bolus injection of gadolinium administered intravenously during ultrafast T2 or T2* acquisitions. The contrast agent

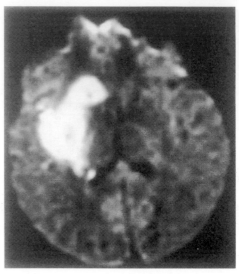

Fig. 20.2 Axial diffusion-weighted image of the brain acquired with a single shot EPI sequence. The high signal intensity represents an area of infarct and restricted diffusion.

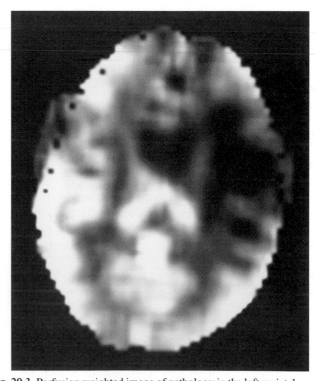

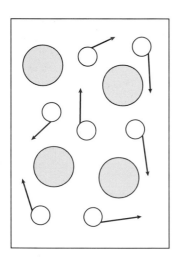 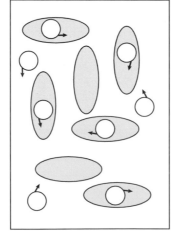

freely diffusing water   restricted water

Fig. 20.1 Free and restricted diffusion of water.

Fig. 20.3 Perfusion weighted image of pathology in the left parietal area.

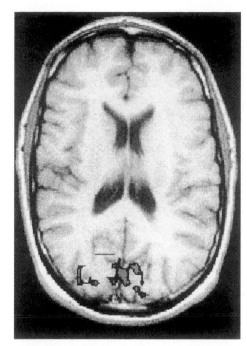

Fig. 20.4 This axial view of the brain was acquired for anatomical information. The irregular area overlaid on the posterior brain is the BOLD acquisition during visual stimulation. Note the increase in signal intensity resulting from increased activity in the visual cortex.

causes transient decreases in T2 and T2* in and around the microvasculature perfused with contrast. After data acquisition, a signal decay curve can be used to ascertain blood volume, transient time and measurement of perfusion. This curve is known as a **time intensity curve**. Time intensity curves for multiple images acquired during and after injection are combined to generate **a cerebral blood volume (CBV) map**. **Mean transit times (MTT)** of contrast through an organ or tissue can also be calculated.

Clinical applications

This is used for evaluation of ischaemic disease or metabolism. On the CBV map, areas of low perfusion appear dark (stroke) whereas areas of higher perfusion appear bright (malignancies).

Functional imaging (fMRI)

Functional MR imaging (fMRI) is a rapid MR imaging technique that acquires images of the brain during activity or stimulus and at rest. The two sets of images are then subtracted demonstrating functional brain activity as the result of increased blood flow to the activated cortex. The most important physiological effect that produces MR signal intensity changes between stimulus and rest is called **blood oxygenation level dependent (BOLD)**. BOLD exploits differences in the magnetic susceptibility of oxyhaemoglobin and deoxyhaemoglobin.

• **Haemoglobin** is a molecule that contains iron and transports oxygen in the vascular system as oxygen binds directly to iron.

• **Oxyhaemoglobin** is a diamagnetic molecule in which the magnetic properties of iron are largely suppressed.

• **Deoxyhaemoglobin** is a paramagnetic molecule that creates an inhomogeneous magnetic field in its immediate vicinity that increases T2*.

At rest, tissue uses a substantial fraction of the blood flowing through the capillaries, so venous blood contains an almost equal mix of oxy- and deoxyhaemoglobin. During exercise however when metabolism is increased, more oxygen is needed and hence more is extracted from the capillaries. The brain is very sensitive to low concentrations of oxyhaemoglobin and therefore the cerebral vascular system increases blood flow to the activated area. This causes a drop in deoxyhaemoglobin that results in a decrease in dephasing and a corresponding increase in signal intensity. Blood oxygenation increases during brain activity and specific locations of the cerebral cortex are activated during specific tasks. For example, seeing activates the visual cortex (Fig. 20.4), hearing the auditory cortex, finger tapping the motor cortex. More sophisticated tasks, including maze paradigms and other thought-provoking tasks, stimulate other brain cortices.

BOLD effects are very short lived and therefore require extremely rapid sequences such as EPI or fast gradient echo. The images are usually acquired with long TEs (40–70 ms) while the task is modulated on and off. The 'off' images are then subtracted from the 'on' images and a more sophisticated statistical analysis is performed. Regions that were activated above some threshold level are overlaid onto anatomic images.

Clinical applications

Primarily development of the understanding of brain function including evaluation of stroke, epilepsy, pain and behavioural problems.

Spectroscopy

Spectroscopy provides a frequency spectrum of a given tissue based on the molecular and chemical structures of that tissue. Peak size and placement within the measured spectrum provide information on how an atom is bonded to a molecule. Most clinical spectroscopy looks at hydrogen but advanced forms are able to evaluate other MR active nuclei. Spatial localization can be achieved by using the **stimulated-echo acquisition mode (STEAM)**. The localized volume is generated via stimulated echoes from spins excited by three 90° RF pulses, and the conventional STEAM sequence detects the stimulated-echo signal. A slice selective RF pulse is applied in conjunction with an X magnetic field gradient. This excites spins in an YZ plane. A 180° slice selective RF pulse is applied in conjunction with a Y magnetic field gradient. This rotates spins located in an XZ plane. A second 180° slice selective RF pulse is applied in conjunction with a Z magnetic field gradient. The second 180° pulse excites spins in an XY plane. The second echo is recorded as the signal. This echo represents the signal from those spins in the intersection of the three planes. Fourier transformation of the echo produces a spectrum of the spins located at the intersection of the three planes.

Clinical applications

Spectroscopy is now becoming a routine part of clinical imaging to evaluate tissue metabolism and identification of tumour types.

21 Gradient functions

Gradients are coils of wire that, when a current is passed through them, alter the magnetic field strength of the magnet in a controlled and predictable way. They add or subtract from the existing field in a linear fashion so that the magnetic field strength at any point along the gradient is known (Fig. 21.1). When a gradient is applied the following occur.

• At **isocentre** the field strength remains unchanged even when the gradient is switched on.

• At a certain distance away from isocentre the field strength either increases or decreases. The magnitude of the change depends on the distance from isocentre and the strength of the gradient.

• The slope of the gradient signifies the rate of change of the magnetic field strength along its length. The **strength** or **amplitude** of the gradient is determined by **how much current** is applied to the gradient coil. Larger currents create steeper gradients so that the change in field strength over distance is greater. The reverse is true of smaller currents (Fig. 21.2).

• The **polarity** of the gradient determines which end of the gradient produces a higher field strength than isocentre (positive) and which a lower field strength than isocentre (negative). The polarity of the gradient is determined by the **direction of the current** flowing through the coil. As the coils are circular, current either flows clockwise or anticlockwise.

• The **maximum amplitude** of the gradient determines the maximum achievable **resolution**.

• The speed with which gradients can be switched on and off are called **the rise time** (Fig. 21.3) and **slew rate**. Both of these factors determine the maximum scan speeds of a system.

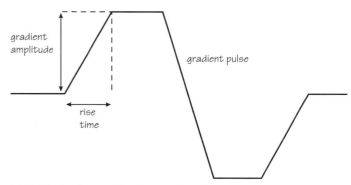

Fig. 21.3 Gradient amplitude versus rise time.

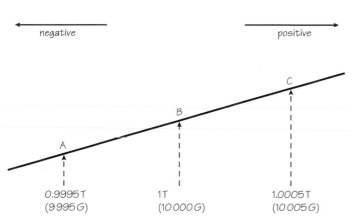

Fig. 21.1 What do you think the precessional frequency will be at A, B and C, if the field strength is 0.5 T and 1.5 T?

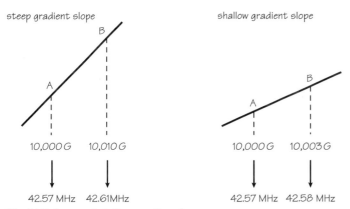

Fig. 21.2 Steep and shallow gradient slopes.

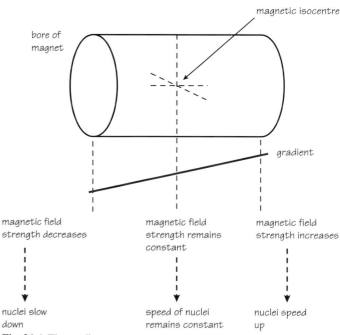

Fig. 21.4 The gradients.

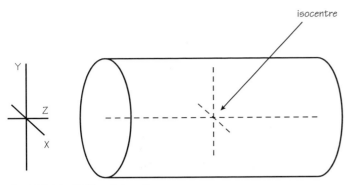

Fig. 21.5 The X, Y and Z gradient axes.

How gradients work

The precessional frequency of the magnetic moments of nuclei is proportional to the magnetic field strength experienced by them (as stated by the Larmor equation). The frequency of the signal received from the patient can be changed according to its position along the gradient. The precessional phase is also affected as faster magnetic moments gain phase compared with their slower neighbours.

Imposing a gradient magnetic field therefore changes:

• the field strength in a linear fashion across a distance in the patient (Fig. 21.4);

• the precessional **frequency** of magnetic moments of nuclei in a linear fashion across a distance in the patient;

• the precessional **phase** of magnetic moments of nuclei in a linear fashion across a distance in the patient.

These characteristics can be used to **encode** the MR signal in three dimensions. In order to do this there must be three orthogonal sets of gradients situated within the bore of the magnet. They are named according to the axis along which they work (Fig. 21.5 and Table 21.1).

The **Z gradient** alters the magnetic field strength along the **Z axis**.

The **Y gradient** alters the magnetic field strength along the **Y axis**.

The **X gradient** alters the magnetic field strength along the **X axis**.

The **isocentre** is the centre of all three gradients. The field strength here does not change even when a gradient is applied.

There are only three gradients but they are used to perform many important functions during a pulse sequence. One of these functions is **spatial encoding**, i.e. spatially locating a signal in three dimensions. In order to do this, three separate functions are necessary. Usually each gradient performs one of the following tasks. The gradient used for each task depends on the plane of the scan and on which gradient the operator selects to perform frequency or phase encoding.

1 Slice selection – locating a slice in the scan plane selected.

2 Spatially locating a signal along the long axis of the image. This is called **frequency encoding**.

3 Spatially locating a signal along the short axis of the image. This is called **phase encoding**.

Table 21.1 Gradient axes in orthogonal imaging.

	Slice selection	Phase encoding	Frequency encoding
Sagittal	X	Y	Z
Axial (body)	Z	Y	X
Axial (head)	Z	X	Y
Coronal	Y	X	Z

22 Slice selection

Mechanism

As a gradient alters the magnetic field strength of the magnet linearly, the magnetic moments of nuclei within a specific slice location along the gradient have a unique precessional frequency when the gradient is on. A slice can therefore be selectively excited by transmitting RF at that unique precessional frequency.

Example: a 1.5 T field strength magnet with a gradient imposed that has changed the field strength by 10 gauss between slice A and B (Fig. 22.1).

- The gradient has changed the field strength by 10 G.
- The precessional frequency of magnetic moments has changed by 100 Hz.
- To excite nuclei in slice A an RF pulse of 67.76 MHz must be applied.
- Slice B and all other slices are not excited because their precessional frequencies are different due to the influence of the gradient.
- To excite slice B, another RF pulse with a frequency of 63.86 MHz must be applied. Nuclei in slice A do not resonate after the application of this pulse because they are spinning at a different frequency.

The scan plane selected determines which gradient performs slice selection (Fig. 22.2).

- The **Z** gradient selects **axial** slices, so that nuclei in the patient's head spin at a different frequency from those in the feet.
- The **Y** gradient selects **coronal** slices, so that nuclei at the back of the patient spin at a different frequency from those at the front.
- The **X** gradient selects **sagittal** slices, so that nuclei on the right-hand side of the patient spin at a different frequency from those on the left.
- A combination of any two gradients selects **oblique** slices.

Slice thickness

In order to attain slice thickness, a range of frequencies must be transmitted to produce resonance across the whole slice (and therefore to excite the whole slice). This range of frequencies is called a **bandwidth** and because RF is being transmitted at this instant, it is specifically called the **transmit bandwidth**.

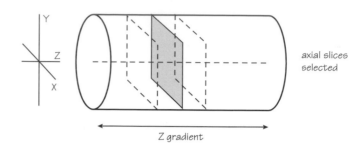

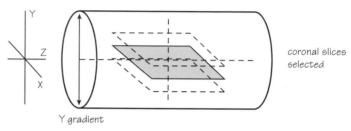

Fig. 22.2 The Y and Z gradients as slice selectors.

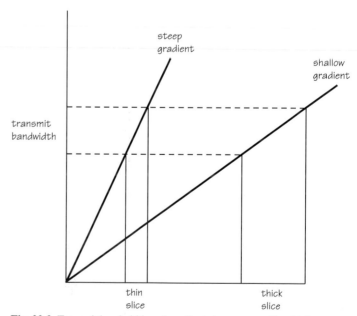

Fig. 22.3 Transmit bandwidth and gradient slope versus slice thickness.

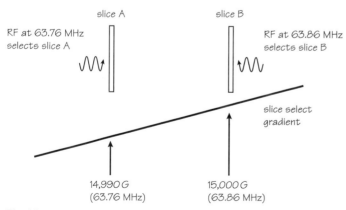

Fig. 22.1 Slice selection.

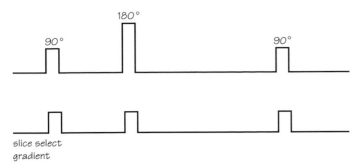

slice select
gradient

Fig. 22.4 The timing of slice selection in spin echo.

• The slice thickness is determined by the slope of the slice select gradient and the transmit bandwidth (Fig. 22.3). It affects in-plane spatial resolution (see Chapter 30).

• **Thin** slices require a **steep** slope and **narrow** transmit bandwidth and improve spatial resolution.

• **Thick** slices require a **shallow** slope and **broad** transmit bandwidth and decrease spatial resolution.

A slice is therefore excited by transmitting RF with a centre frequency corresponding to the middle of the slice and a bandwidth and gradient slope according to the thickness of the slice required. The **slice gap** or **skip** is the space between slices. Too small a gap in relation to the slice thickness can lead to an artefact called cross excitation.

The slice select gradient is switched on during the delivery of the RF excitation pulse (Fig. 22.4). It is switched on for 3.2 ms in the positive direction. The slice select gradient is also switched on during the 180° pulse in spin echo sequences so that the rephasing pulse can be delivered specifically to the selected slice.

23 Phase encoding

After a slice has been selected, the magnetic field strength experienced by nuclei within the excited slice equals the field strength of the system. The precessional frequencies of spins within the slice is equal to the Larmor frequency. The frequency of the signal from the slice also equals the Larmor frequency, regardless of the location of each signal. The system has to use gradients to gain two-dimensional information representing the spatial location of the spins within the slice. When a gradient is switched on, the precessional frequency of a nucleus is determined by its physical location on the gradient.

Mechanism

The gradient also changes the **phase** of the magnetic moment of each nucleus. The phase of a magnetic moment is its place on the 'cone' or

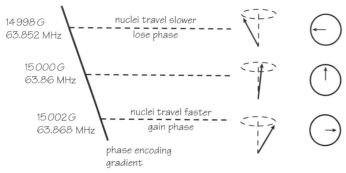

14 998 G
63.852 MHz

nuclei travel slower
lose phase

15 000 G
63.86 MHz

15 002 G
63.868 MHz

nuclei travel faster
gain phase

phase encoding
gradient

Fig. 23.1 Phase shift.

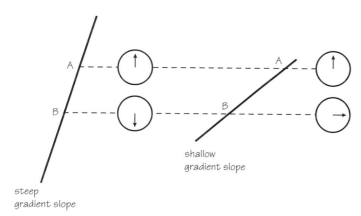

A

B

shallow
gradient slope

steep
gradient slope

Fig. 23.2 The relationship between phase encoding gradient slope and phase shift.

precessional path at any moment in time. It can be compared to the position of the little hand on a clock.

• A nucleus that experiences a higher magnetic field strength when the gradient is switched on, gains phase relative to its position without the gradient on. This is because when a spin precesses at a higher frequency it is travelling faster and therefore moves further around 'the clock' than it would have done with the gradient off.

• If a nucleus experiences a lower magnetic field strength with the gradient on, its magnetic moment slows down relative to its speed or frequency with the gradient off and loses phase. Therefore, the presence of a gradient along one axis of the image causes a **phase shift** of nuclei along the length of the gradient (Fig. 23.1). The degree of phase shift relative to isocentre depends on its distance from isocentre.

• To locate signal along the shortest dimension of anatomy in the image, a phase encoding gradient is applied which produces a phase shift of spins along the gradient.

• When the gradient is switched off, nuclei return to the Larmor frequency but their phase shift remains, i.e. they all travel at the same speed around the clock but their positions on the clock are different. This phase shift is used to locate the nuclei (and therefore signal) spatially along one dimension of the image.

• The **slope** or amplitude of the phase encoding gradient determines the degree of phase shift (Fig. 23.2). Steeper gradients produce a greater phase shift between two points than shallower gradients. Steeper gradients increase the **phase matrix** of the **field of view (FOV)** (see Chapter 30) and therefore the resolution of the image along the phase axis or dimension of the FOV.

The phase encoding gradient is switched on after the RF excitation pulse has been switched off. It is normally turned on for 4 ms and the amplitude and polarity of the gradient is altered for each phase encoding step (Fig. 23.3).

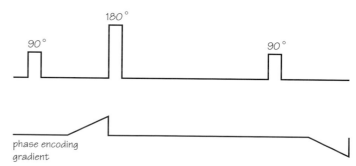

90°

180°

90°

phase encoding
gradient

Fig. 23.3 The timing of phase encoding in spin echo.

24 Frequency encoding

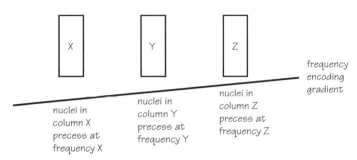

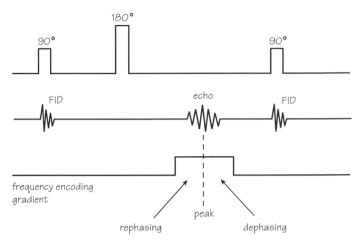

Fig. 24.1 Frequency shift.

Fig. 24.2 The timing of frequency encoding in spin echo.

After a slice has been selected, the magnetic field strength experienced by nuclei within the excited slice equals the field strength of the system. The precessional frequencies of spins within the slice is equal to the Larmor frequency. The frequency of the signal from the slice also equals the Larmor frequency, regardless of the location of each signal. The system has to use gradients to gain two-dimensional information representing the spatial location of the spins within the slice. When a gradient is switched on, the precessional frequency of a nucleus is determined by its physical location on the gradient (Fig. 24.1).

Mechanism

A gradient corresponding to the long axis dimension of anatomy in the image is switched on to locate signal along this axis. The frequency change caused by the gradient is used to locate each signal. It produces a **frequency change** or **frequency shift** in the following manner.
• The spins of nuclei experiencing a higher magnetic field strength due to the gradient speed up, i.e. their precessional frequencies increase.
• The spins of nuclei experiencing a lower magnetic field strength due

to the presence of the gradient slow down, i.e. their precessional frequencies decrease.
• This is called **frequency encoding** and results in a **frequency shift** of nuclei (and therefore signal) relative to their position on the gradient.
• The **frequency encoding gradient** is switched on during the echo (Fig. 24.2). It is often called the **readout** gradient because, during its application, frequencies within the signal are read by the system. The gradient is normally switched on for 8 ms and the echo is usually centred to the middle of the gradient application. The readout gradient is switched on in the positive direction.
• The **slope** of the frequency encoding gradient determines the **size of the FOV** and therefore the image resolution.

25 K space characteristics

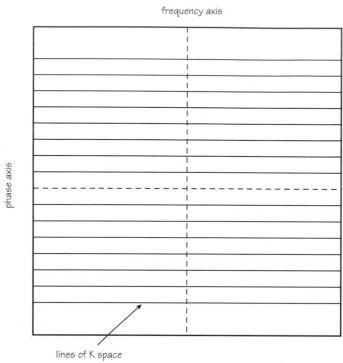

Fig. 25.1 K space.

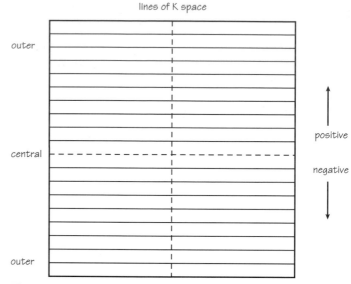

Fig. 25.2 The two halves of K space.

K space is an area where data collected from the signal are stored. It is a spatial frequency domain, i.e. where information about the frequency of a signal and where it comes from in the patient is collected and stored. As frequency is defined as phase change per unit time and is measured in radians – the unit of K space is radians per cm. K space does not correspond to the image, i.e. the top of K space does not correspond with the top of the image. K space is merely an area where data are stored until the scan is over.

K space is rectangular and has two axes (Fig. 25.1):
• the **frequency axis** of K space that is centred in the middle of the K space perpendicular to the phase axis; and
• the phase axis of K space that is centred in the middle of a series of horizontal **lines**, the number of which corresponds to the number of phase encodings performed (**phase matrix**).

Every time a frequency or phase encoding is performed, data are collected and stored in a line of K space. The lines **nearest** to the phase axis both positively and negatively, are called the **central** lines (Fig. 25.2). The lines **farthest** from the phase axis, both positively and negatively, are called the **outer** lines. The top half of K space is termed **positive** and the bottom half of K space is termed **negative**.

The polarity of the phase gradient determines whether the positive or negative half of K space is filled. Positive gradient slopes fill lines in the positive half of K space, and negative gradients fill lines in the negative half.

Lines are numbered relative to the central horizontal axis, starting from the centre and moving out towards the outer areas of K space.

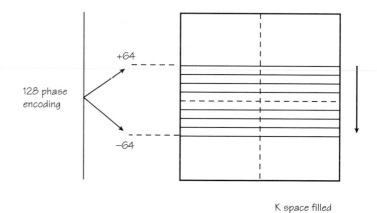

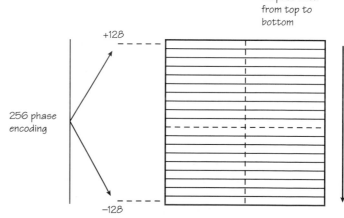

Fig. 25.3 K space filling.

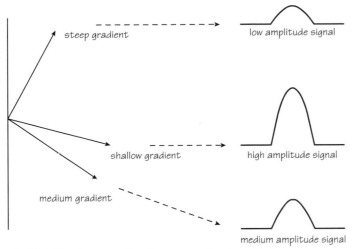

Fig. 25.4 The phase encoding slope versus signal amplitude.

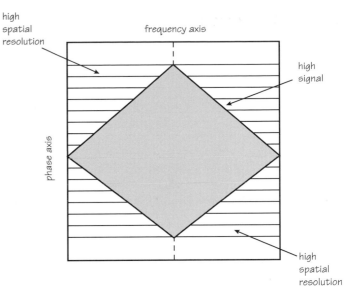

Fig. 25.5 K space – SNR and spatial resolution.

Lines in the top half are labelled positive, those in the bottom half, negative. The central lines of K space are always filled regardless of the phase matrix. For example, if 128 phase matrix is required, lines +64 to −64 are filled rather than lines +128 to 0. K space lines are usually filled linearly, i.e. either from top to bottom, or from bottom to top (Fig. 25.3).

K space is symmetrical about both axes, i.e. data in the right hand side of K space are identical to those on the left, and data in the top half are identical to those in the bottom half. This is called **conjugate symmetry**.

K space filling and signal amplitude
Phase axis

The **central** lines of K space are filled with data produced after the application of **shallow** phase encoding gradient slopes. The **outer** lines of K space are filled with data produced after the application of the **steep** phase encoding gradient slopes. The lines in-between the central and outer portions are filled with the intermediate phase encoding slopes.

Shallow phase encoding slopes do not produce a large phase shift along their axis. Therefore rephasing of magnetic moments by an RF pulse or a gradient is more efficient, as the inherent phase shift after phase encoding is small. **The resultant signal therefore has a large amplitude** (Fig. 25.4).

Steep phase encoding slopes produce a large phase shift along their axis. Therefore rephasing of magnetic moments is less efficient because the inherent phase shift after phase encoding is great. **The resultant signal has a small amplitude** (Fig. 25.4).

Frequency axis

Frequencies sampled from the signal are mapped into K space relative to the frequency axis. The centre of the echo represents the maximum signal amplitude as all the magnetic moments are in phase at this point, whereas magnetic moments are either rephasing or dephasing on either side of the peak of the echo, and therefore the signal amplitude here is less. The amplitude of frequencies sampled is mapped relative to the frequency axis, so that the centre of the echo is placed central to the frequency axis. The rephasing and dephasing portions of the echo are mapped to the left and the right of the frequency axis.

K space filling and spatial resolution
Phase axis

The outer lines of K space contain data produced after steep phase encoding gradient slopes, and are only filled when many phase encodings have been performed. The number of phase encodings performed determines the number of pixels in the FOV along the phase encoding axis. When a large number of phase encodings are performed, there are more pixels in the FOV along the phase axis and therefore each pixel is smaller. If the FOV is fixed, pixels of smaller dimensions result in an image with a high spatial resolution, i.e. two points within the image can be distinguished more easily when the pixels are small (see Chapter 30). In addition, as the amplitude of the phase encoding gradient slope increases, the degree of phase shift along the gradient also increases. Two points adjacent to each other have a different phase value and can therefore be differentiated from each other. Therefore data collected after steep phase encoding gradient slopes produce greater spatial resolution in the image.

Summary

• The outer lines of K space contain data with a high spatial resolution as they are filled by steep phase encoding gradient slopes (Fig. 25.5).
• The central lines of K space contain data with a low spatial resolution as they are filled by shallow phase encoding gradient slopes.
• The central portion of K space contains data that have high signal amplitude and low spatial resolution.
• The outer portion of K space contains data that have high spatial resolution and low signal amplitude.

26 Data acquisition

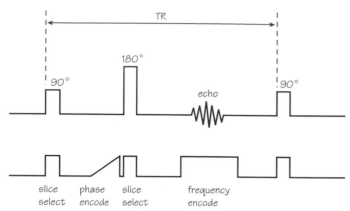

Fig. 26.1 Gradient timing in spin echo.

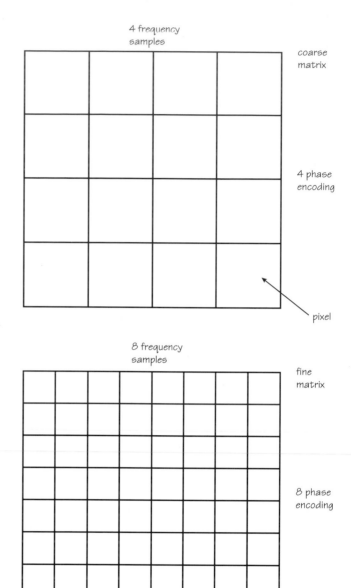

Fig. 26.2 The image matrix.

As a result of spatial encoding, the spins are phase shifted along one axis of the image and frequency shifted along the other. The system can now tell the individual spins apart by the number of times they pass across the receiver coil (frequency) and their position in the cycle as they do so (phase). Each of the gradients is switched on at a particular time in the pulse sequence and for a certain length of time (see Chapters 23 and 24) (Fig. 26.1).

Each system has a minimum length of time required to switch all three gradients on and off. The speed with which it can do this depends on the sophistication of the gradients, their amplifiers and switching mechanisms. Whatever a system's characteristics, it cannot receive an echo until it has performed all these gradient functions. In practice this means that the minimum TE is sometimes limited.

Image production

The information obtained from the encoding process now has to be translated onto the image. The image consists of a **field of view (FOV)** that relates to the amount of anatomy covered. The FOV can be square or rectangular and is divided up into **pixels** or picture elements (Fig. 26.2). The pixels exist within a two dimensional grid or **matrix** into which the system maps each individual signal.

The number of pixels within the FOV depends on the number of frequency samples and phase encodings performed. The matrix size is annotated by two figures, one usually corresponding to the number of frequency samples (data points), the second to the number of phase encodings performed.

Each pixel is allocated a signal intensity, depending on the signal amplitude, with a distinct frequency and phase shift value. This is performed via by a mathematical process known as **Fast Fourier Transform (FFT)** (Fig. 26.3). In its raw data form, the frequency of each signal is plotted against time, i.e. the signal is measured in relation to its amplitude over a period of time. During FFT the system converts this raw data so that the signal amplitude is measured relative to its frequency. This enables the creation of an image, where each pixel is allo-

cated a signal intensity corresponding to the amplitude of signal originating from the anatomy at the position of each pixel in the matrix.

Data acquisition and frequency encoding

The application of RF excitation pulses and gradients produces a range of different frequencies within the signal. All of these frequencies must be sampled by the system in order to produce an accurate image from the data. The range of frequencies sampled and encoded within the FOV is called the **receive bandwidth** (Fig. 26.4). The magnitude of the

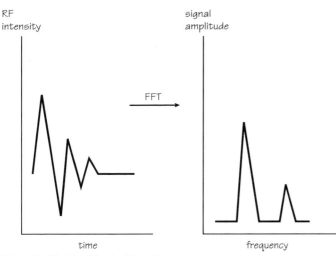

Fig. 26.3 The Fast Fourier Transform.

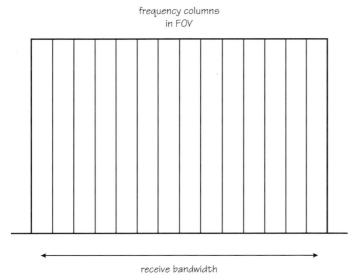

frequency columns
in FOV

receive bandwidth

Fig. 26.4 Frequencies sampled are mapped across the FOV.

frequency encoding gradient, along with the receive bandwidth, determines the size of the FOV, i.e. the distance across the patient into which the frequencies within the receive bandwidth must fit.

FOV 24 cm   BandW 32 000 Hz   32 000 Hz must be mapped across 24 cm.

FOV 12 cm   BandW 32 000 Hz   32 000 Hz must be mapped across 12 cm.

Every time a frequency is sampled, data from it are stored in a line of K space. This is called a **data point**. The number of data points in each line of K space corresponds to the frequency matrix (either 256, 512 or 1024 on most systems).

After the scan is over, the computer looks at the data points in K space and mathematically converts information in each data point into a frequency. From this the image is formed. As the frequency encoding gradient is always applied during the sampling of data from the echo, it is often called the **readout gradient** (although the gradient is not collecting the data, the computer is doing this).

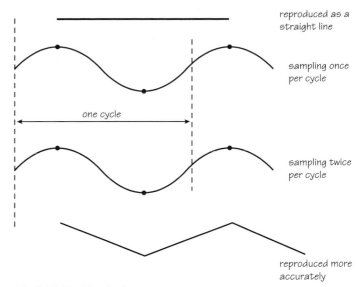

reproduced as a straight line

sampling once per cycle

one cycle

sampling twice per cycle

reproduced more accurately

Fig. 26.5 The Nyquist theorem.

• The time available to the system to sample frequencies in the signal is called the **sampling time**.
• The rate at which frequencies are sampled is called the **sampling rate**.
• The sampling rate is determined by the **Nyquist theorem** (Fig. 26.5) that states that the sampling rate must be at least twice the frequency of the highest frequency in the echo. If this does not occur, data points collected in K space do not accurately reflect all frequencies present in the signal.

In order to produce an accurate image, the frequency derived from the data points must look like the original frequencies in the signal. If the sampling rate frequency only matches the highest frequency present in the echo, only one data point is collected per cycle. This means that there is insufficient data to reproduce all the original frequencies accurately. If the sampling rate frequency obeys the Nyquist theorem and samples at twice the highest frequency in the echo, then there will be sufficient data points to reproduce the original frequencies accurately.

There is a relationship between the receive bandwidth and the frequency matrix selected. Enough data points must be collected to achieve the required frequency matrix with a particular receive bandwidth.

Changing the receive bandwidth

Frequency matrix 256

If the frequency matrix is 256, then 256 data points must be collected and laid out in each line of K space. The number of frequencies that occur during the sampling time is determined by the receive bandwidth. To satisfy the Nyquist theorem, 128 frequencies must occur during the sampling time.

For example:

Receive bandwidth 32 000 Hz (32 000 cycles/s)

    sampling time = 8 ms, therefore 128 cycles occur in 8 ms

    sampling rate = 2 × 128 = 256

    256 data points collected = frequency matrix 256

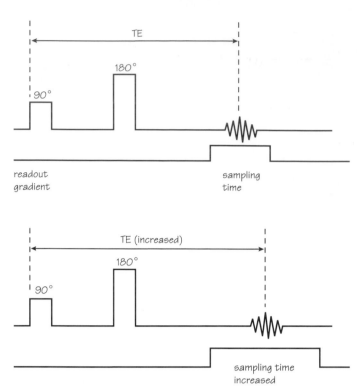

Fig. 26.6 The sampling time and the TE.

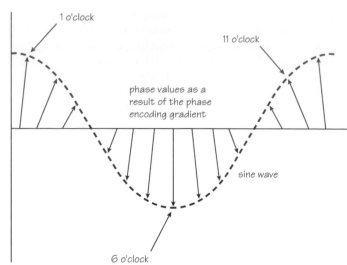

Fig. 26.7 The sine wave.

Receive bandwidth 16 000 Hz (16 000 cycles/s)

> sampling time = 8 ms, therefore 64 cycles occur in 8 ms
>
> sampling rate = 2 × 64 = 128
>
> 128 data points collected

Therefore, if the receive bandwidth is reduced without altering any other parameter, there are insufficient data points to produce a 256 frequency matrix.

As the sampling rate is not changed, the sampling time must be increased to collect the necessary 256 points. As the echo is usually centred in the middle of the sampling window, the minimum TE increases as the sampling time increases (Fig. 26.6).

Changing the frequency matrix

Frequency matrix 512

If the frequency matrix is 512, then 512 data points must be collected and laid out in each line of K space. The number of frequencies that occur during the sampling time is determined by the receive bandwidth. To satisfy the Nyquist theorem, 256 frequencies must occur during the sampling time.

For example:

Receive bandwidth 32 000 Hz (32 000 cycles/s)

> sampling time = 8 ms, therefore 128 cycles occur in 8 ms
>
> sampling rate = 2 × 128 = 256
>
> 256 data points collected = frequency matrix 256

Therefore, if the frequency matrix is increased without altering any other parameter, there are insufficient data points to produce a 512 frequency matrix.

As the sampling rate is not changed, the sampling time must be increased to permit 256 cycles to be sampled during the sampling window. As the echo is usually centred in the middle of the sampling window, the minimum TE increases as the sampling time increases.

Therefore either increasing the frequency matrix or reducing the receive bandwidth increases the minimum TE.

Data acquisition and phase encoding

A certain value of phase shift is also obtained according to the slope of the phase encoding gradient. The slope of the phase encoding gradient determines which line of K space is filled with the data from that frequency and phase encoding. In order to fill out different lines of K space, the slope of the phase encoding gradient is altered after each TR. If the slope of the phase encoding gradient is not altered, the same line of K space is filled in all the time. In order to finish the scan or acquisition, all the selected lines of K space must be filled. The number of lines of K space that are filled is determined by the number of different phase encoding slopes that are applied:

- 128 different phase encoding slopes selected, 128 lines of K space are filled to complete the scan;
- 256 different phase encoding slopes selected, 256 lines of K space are filled to complete the scan.

The slope of the phase encoding gradient determines the magnitude of the phase shift between two points in the patient. **Steep** slopes produce a **large phase difference** between two points, whereas **shallow** slopes produce **small phase shifts** between the same two points.

The system cannot measure phase directly; it can only measure frequency. The system therefore converts the phase shift into frequency by creating a sine wave formed by combining all the phase values associated with a certain phase shift (Fig. 26.7). This sine wave has a certain frequency or pseudo-frequency (as it has been indirectly obtained).

In order to fill a different line of K space, a different pseudo-frequency must be obtained. If a different pseudo-frequency is not obtained, the same line of K space is filled over and over again. To create a different pseudo-frequency, a different phase shift must be produced by the phase encoding gradient (Fig. 26.8). The phase encoding gradient is therefore switched on to a different amplitude or slope to produce a different phase shift value. Therefore, the change in phase shift created by the altered phase encoding gradient slope results in a sine wave with a different pseudo-frequency. Every TR, each slice is frequency encoded (resulting in the same frequency shift), and phase encoded with a different slope of phase encoding gradient to produce a different pseudo-frequency. Once all the lines of selected K space have been filled, acquisition of data is complete and the scan is over. The acquired data held in K space are now converted into an image via FFT.

Data acquisition and scan time

In conventional data acquisition:

$$\text{scan time} = \text{TR} \times \text{phase matrix} \times \text{number of signal averages (NSA/NEX)}$$

TR

Every TR, each slice is frequency encoded (resulting in the same frequency shift), and phase encoded with a different slope of phase encoding gradient to produce a different pseudo-frequency. Different lines in K space are filled after every TR. Once all the lines of selected K space have been filled, acquisition of data is complete and the scan is over.

Phase matrix

The phase encoding gradient slope is altered every TR and is applied to each selected slice in order to phase encode it. At each phase encode a different line of K space is filled (Fig. 26.9). The number of phase encoding steps therefore affects the length of the scan.

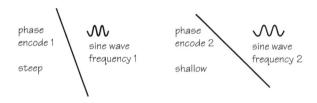

Fig. 26.8 Phase encoding slope versus pseudo-frequency.

K space

line 1	frequency/phase data	phase encode 1
line 2	frequency/phase data	phase encode 2
line 3	frequency/phase data	phase encode 3
line 4	frequency/phase data	phase encode 4
line 5	frequency/phase data	phase encode 5

to 128, 192, ... 512 phase encodes

Fig. 26.9 K space lines.

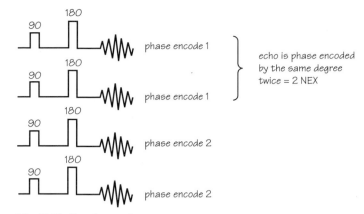

Fig. 26.10 Signal averaging.

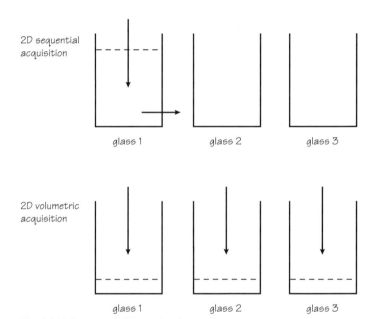

Fig. 26.11 Data acquisition – the glass analogy.

- For **128** phase encodings selected, **128 lines** are filled.
- For **256** phase encodings selected, **256 lines** are filled.
- As one phase encoding is performed each TR (to each slice): **128** phase encodings requires **128 × TR** to complete the scan, **256** phase encodings requires **256 × TR** to complete the scan.
- If the TR is 1 s (1000 ms) the scan takes 128 s (if 128 phase encodings are performed) and 256 s (if 256 phase encodings are performed).

Number of signal averages (NSA/NEX)

The signal can be sampled more than once with the same slope of phase encoding gradient. Doing so will fill each line of K space more than once. The number of times each signal is sampled with the same slope of phase encoding gradient is usually called the **number of signal averages (NSA)** or the **number of excitations (NEX)** (Fig. 26.10). The higher the NEX, the more data that are stored in each line of K space. As there are more data stored in each line of K space, the amplitude of signal at each frequency and phase shift is greater.

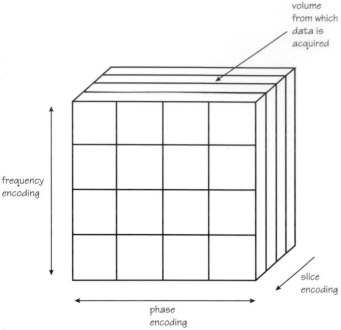

volume
from which
data is
acquired

frequency
encoding

slice
encoding

phase
encoding

Fig. 26.12 Encoding in a volume acquisition.

Types of acquisition

Three-dimensional volumetric sequential acquisitions acquire all the data from slice 1 and then go on to acquire all the data from slice 2 (all the lines in K space are filled for slice 1 and then all the lines of K space are filled for slice 2, etc.). The slices are therefore displayed as they are acquired.

Two-dimensional volumetric acquisitions fill one line of K space for slice 1, and then go on to to fill the same line of K space for slice 2, etc. When this line has been filled for all the slices, the next line of K space is filled for slices 1, 2, 3, etc. (Fig. 26.11).

Three-dimensional volumetric acquisition (volume imaging) acquires data from an entire volume of tissue, rather than in separate slices (Fig. 26.12). The excitation pulse is not slice selective, and the whole prescribed imaging volume is excited. At the end of the acquisition the volume or slab is divided into discrete locations or partitions by the slice select gradient that, when switched on, separates the slices according to their phase value along the gradient. This process is called **slice encoding**. Many slices can be obtained (typically 28, 64 or 128) without a slice gap.

27 K space traversal

The way in which K space is traversed and filled depends on a combination of the polarity and amplitude of both the frequency and phase encoding gradients.

• The amplitude of the **frequency** encoding gradient determines how far to **the left and right** K space is traversed and this in turn determines the size of the FOV in the frequency direction of the image.

• The amplitude of the **phase** encoding gradient determines how far **up and down** K space is filled and in turn determines the size of the FOV in the phase direction of the image (or the spatial resolution when the FOV is square).

The polarity of each gradient defines the direction travelled through K space as follows:

• **frequency** encoding gradient **positive**, K space traversed **from left to right**;

• **frequency** encoding gradient **negative**, K space traversed **from right to left**;

• **phase** encoding gradient **positive**, fills **top** half of K space;

• **phase** encoding gradient **negative**, fills **bottom** half of K space

K space traversal in gradient echo

In a gradient echo sequence the frequency encoding gradient switches negatively to dephase the FID and then positively to rephase and produce a gradient echo.

• When the frequency encoding gradient is negative, K space is traversed from right to left. The starting point of K space filling is always at the centre, so K space is initially traversed from the centre to the left, to a distance (*A*) that depends on the amplitude of the negative lobe of the frequency encoding gradient (Fig. 27.1).

• The phase encode in this example is positive and therefore a line in the top half of K space is filled. The amplitude of this gradient determines the distance travelled (*B*). The larger the amplitude of the phase gradient, the higher up in K space the line that is filled with data from the echo. Therefore the combination of the phase gradient and the negative lobe of the frequency gradient determines at what point in K space data storage begins.

• The frequency encoding gradient is then switched positively and during its application data is read from the echo. As the frequency encoding gradient is positive, data is placed in a line of K space from left to right. The distance travelled depends on the amplitude of the positive lobe of the gradient which in turn determines the size of the FOV.

• If the phase gradient is negative then a line in the bottom half of K space is filled in exactly the same manner.

K space traversal in spin echo

K space traversal in spin echo sequences is more complex as the 180° RF pulse affects K space traversal dramatically. It causes the point to which K space has been traversed to be flipped to the mirror point on the opposite side of K space. Therefore, in spin echo the gradient configurations necessary to reach the left side of K space and begin data collection are different.

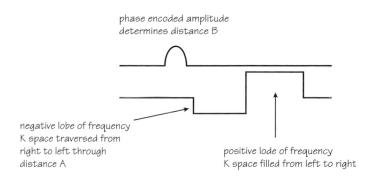

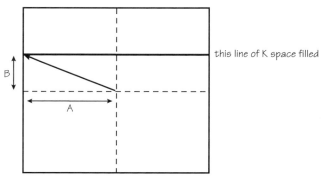

Fig. 27.1 K space traversal in gradient echo imaging.

K space traversal in single shot

Filling K space in single shot imaging involves rapidly switching the frequency encoding gradient from positive to negative; positively to fill a line of K space from left to right and negatively to fill a line from right to left. As the frequency encoding gradient switches its polarity so rapidly it is said to oscillate.

The phase gradient also has to switch on and off rapidly but its polarity does not need to change in this type of K space traversal. The first application of the phase gradient is maximum positive to fill the top line. The next application (to encode the next echo) is still positive but its amplitude is slightly less so that the next line down is filled. This process is repeated until the centre of K space is reached when the phase gradient switches negatively to fill the bottom lines. The amplitude is gradually increased until maximum negative polarity is achieved filling the bottom line of K space. This type of gradient switching is called **blipping** (Fig. 27.2).

K space traversal in spiral imaging

A more complex type of K space traversal is spiral (Fig. 27.3). In this example both the readout and the phase gradient switch their polarity rapidly and oscillate. In this spiral form of K space traversal, not only does the frequency encoding gradient oscillate to fill lines from left to right and then right to left, but as K space filling begins at the centre, the phase gradient must also oscillate to fill a line in the top half followed by a line in the bottom half.

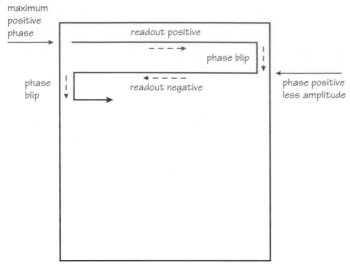

Fig. 27.2 Oscillation of frequency, blipping of phase.

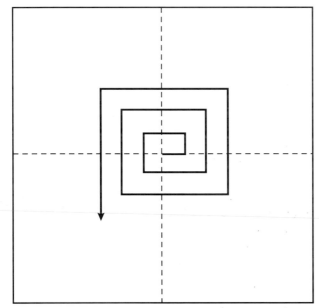

Fig. 27.3 Spiral K space traversal in EPI.

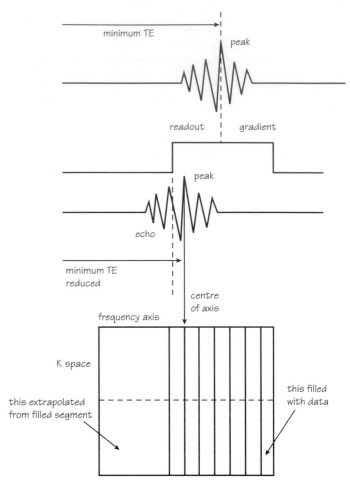

Fig. 27.4 Partial echo.

Alternative K space filling techniques
Partial or fractional echo imaging
• Partial echo imaging (Fig. 27.4) exploits the conjugate symmetry of K space. It is performed when only part of the signal is read by the frequency encoding gradient.

• As the peak of the echo or signal is usually centred in the middle of the sampling time, the signal is mapped relative to the frequency axis of K space and one half of the frequency area of K space is the mirror image of the other half. Therefore, data placed in one half of the frequency area of K space look exactly like that in the other half.

• If only frequencies in one half of the echo are sampled, only half of the frequency area of K space is filled. However, as the remaining is a mirror image, the system can calculate its amplitude accordingly. The echo no longer has to be centred on the middle of the frequency encoding gradient, as it can now occur at the beginning of the frequency

encoding gradient application. As the peak of the echo occurs closer to the RF excitation pulse, the TE can be reduced.

Partial or fractional averaging
• Partial averaging exploits the symmetry of K space (Fig. 27.5). The negative and positive halves of K space on either side of the phase axis are symmetrical and a mirror image of each other. As long as at least half of the lines of K space that have been selected are filled during the acquisition, the system has enough data to produce an image.

• If only 60% of K space is filled, only 60% of the phase encodings selected need to be performed to complete the scan, and the remaining lines are filled with zeros. The scan time is therefore reduced but fewer data are acquired so the image has less signal.

Rectangular FOV (see Chapter 30)
• The incremental step between each line of K space is inversely proportional to the FOV in the phase direction.

• The outermost lines of K space are filled to maintain resolution (256 × 256, +/− 128 lines filled). The incremental step between each line is doubled (only 128 lines filled instead of 256) (Fig. 27.6).

• The scan time is halved as only 128 lines filled.

• The size of the FOV in the phase direction is halved.

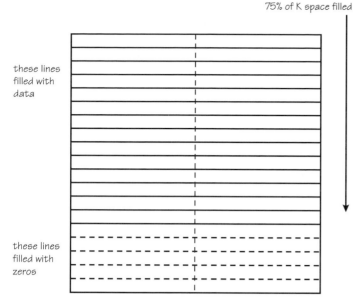

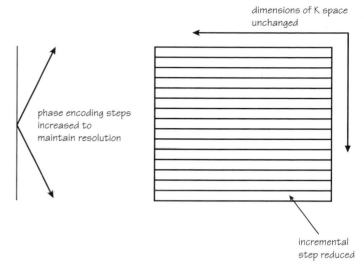

Fig. 27.5 Partial averaging.

Fig. 27.7 Anti-aliasing (phase) and K space filling.

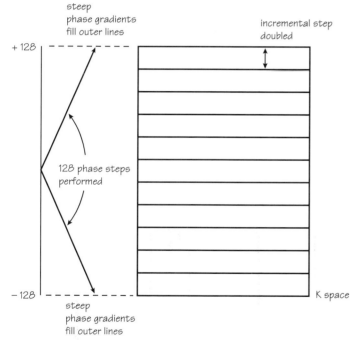

Fig. 27.6 Rectangular FOV and K space filling.

Anti-aliasing/oversampling (see Chapter 36)
• The incremental step between each line of K space is inversely proportional to the FOV in the phase direction.
• The outermost lines of K space are filled to maintain resolution (256 × 256, +/− 128 lines filled). The incremental step between each line is halved (only 512 lines filled instead of 256) (Fig. 27.7).
• Oversampling of data occurs so there is no phase duplication between anatomy outside the FOV and that inside the FOV.

• The NSA/NEX is usually halved to maintain the scan time.
• The size of the FOV in the phase direction is doubled but the outer portions are discarded.

Fast spin echo (See Chapter 13)
In fast spin echo multiple lines of K space are filled per TR so shortening the scan time as K space is filled more efficiently. The number of lines filled per TR is called the turbo factor or echo train length (ETL or turbo factor). Central lines are filled around the effective TE to weight the image correctly.

Single shot
In single shot techniques, K space is filled in one go by rapidly switching the phase and/or frequency encoding gradients. In single shot techniques there is no repetition so TR equals infinity. K space is filled either from top to bottom (frequency oscillates, phase blips) or spirally from the centre out (frequency and phase oscillate in resonance).

Segmented
In segmented K space filling, K space is filled in segments, either in two halves or four quarters. This is achieved by having long ETLs or turbo factors such as 128 or 64. It enables rapid acquisitions with fewer artefacts than single shot imaging.

Key hole
In key hole techniques all of K space is only filled in the first TR (i.e. lines +/− 64). After the first TR only the central lines are filled during acquisition to give signal. Resolution is determined by the outer lines that are only filled during the first TR.

Respiratory compensation (ROPE)
The system ascertains when chest wall motion is high from bellows attached to the patient's chest. Central lines, that give the highest signal, are filled when the chest wall is stationary. Most of the data in the signal are therefore acquired when the chest is still.

28 Signal-to-noise ratio (SNR)

The **signal-to-noise** ratio is defined as the ratio of the amplitude of the MR signal to the amplitude of the background noise. The **MR signal** is the voltage induced in the receiver coil by the precession of the NMV in the transverse plane. It occurs at specific frequencies and time intervals (TE). **Noise** is the undesired signal resulting from the MR system, the environment and the patient. It occurs at all frequencies and randomly in time. To increase the SNR usually requires increasing the signal relative to the noise. Parameters that affect SNR are field strength, proton density, coil type and position, TR, TE, flip angle, number of signal averages and receive bandwidth.

Field strength

The signal-to-noise ratio is affected by the strength of the magnet. At higher field strengths there are more spin up than spin down nuclei as fewer have enough energy to oppose the increased field (see Chapter 3). As a result the NMV increases thereby increasing the available signal.

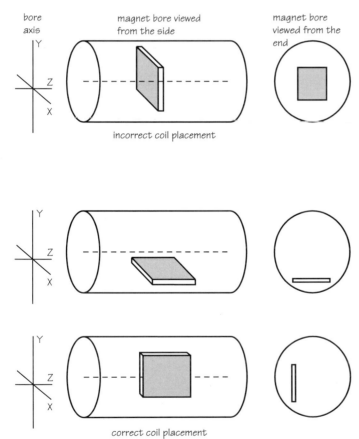

Fig. 28.1 Correct placement of a flat surface coil in the bore of the magnet. The surface of the coil (shaded) area must be parallel to the Z axis to receive signal. The coil is therefore positioned so that transverse magnetization created in the X and Y axes is perpendicular to the coil.

Proton density

Structures like the pelvis contain tissues that have a high proton density such as fat, muscle and bone. Others, such as the chest, contain mainly air-filled lung spaces, vessels and very little dense tissue. When scanning areas with a low proton density it is likely that measures to boost the SNR will be required. This may result in an increase in scan time.

Coil type and position

Small coils like the neck coil provide good local SNR but have a small coverage. Large coils such as the body coil provide much larger coverage but result in lower SNR. A good compromise is to use a phased array coil that uses multiple small coils that provide good SNR and the data from these are combined to produce an image with good coverage.

The positioning of the receiver coil is also very important. In order to receive the maximum signal, receiver coils must be placed in the transverse plane perpendicular to the main field. In a superconducting system this means placing the coil either over, under, or to the right or left of the area being examined. Orientation of the coil perpendicular to the table as in the upper diagram in Fig. 28.1 results in zero signal generation.

TR

The TR determines how much longitudinal magnetization recovers between excitation pulses and how much is available to be flipped into the transverse plane. At very short TRs, very little longitudinal magnetization recovers so only a small amount of transverse magnetization is created and therefore results in an image with poor SNR. Increasing the TR improves the SNR as more longitudinal magnetization, and therefore more transverse magnetization, is created. Although short TRs are required for T1 weighting, reducing this parameter too much may severely compromise the SNR.

TE

The TE determines how much dephasing of transverse magnetization occurs between the excitation pulse and the echo. At short TEs, as very little transverse magnetization has dephased, the signal amplitude and therefore the SNR of the image is high. Increasing the TE reduces the SNR as more transverse magnetization dephases (Fig. 28.2). Although long TEs are required for T2 weighting, increasing this parameter too much compromises the SNR.

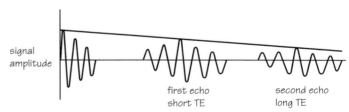

Fig. 28.2 TE versus SNR.

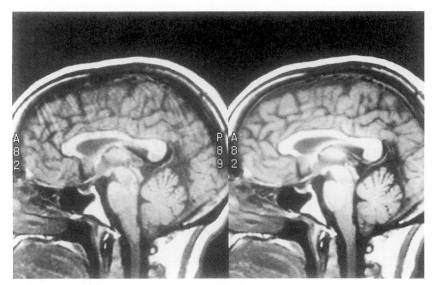

Fig. 28.3 Sagittal images of the brain. The image on the left used partial averaging and took 56 s to acquire. The image on the right, used four signal averages and took 6 min to acquire (all other parameters remained constant). The image on the right has a greater SNR than that on the left.

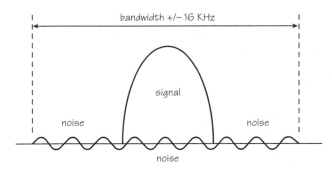

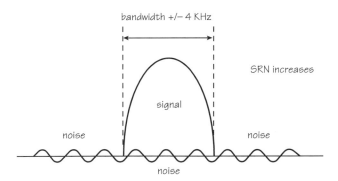

Fig. 28.4 Bandwidth versus SNR.

Flip angle

The size of the flip angle determines how much longitudinal magnetization is converted into transverse magnetization by the excitation pulse. With a large flip angle all available longitudinal magnetization is converted into transverse magnetization and hence maximum signal amplitude, whereas with small flip angles only a proportion of the longitudinal magnetization is converted to transverse magnetization (see

Fig. 15.1). The flip angle is commonly varied in gradient echo sequences where a low flip angle is required for T2* and proton density weighted imaging (see Chapter 15). However they also result in images with low SNR and hence measures may have to be taken to improve it.

Number of signal averages (NSA/NEX)

This parameter determines the number of times frequencies in the signal are sampled with the same slope of phase encoding gradient. Increasing the NEX increases the signal collected. However, noise is also sampled. As noise occurs at all frequencies and randomly, doubling the number of signal averages only increases the SNR by a square root of two. Because of this relationship the benefits of increasing the SNR as the number of signal averages increases are reduced but the scan times increase proportionally.

The images in Fig. 28.3 were acquired with one signal average (on the left) as compared with the image (on the right) acquired with four signal averages. Although the right-hand image has better SNR the difference is not significant. In addition, the right-hand image took four times longer to acquire than the left-hand image. Look carefully at the image on the left and the motion artefact from pulsation of blood in the superior sagittal sinus. Why is this reduced in the image on the right?

Receive bandwidth

This is the range of frequencies sampled during readout. Reducing the receive bandwidth reduces the proportion of noise sampled relative to signal (Fig. 28.4). Reducing the receive bandwidth is a very effective way of boosting the SNR. However, reducing the bandwidth increases:
• the minimum TE, so this technique is not suitable for T1 or PD imaging;
• an artefact known as chemical shift (*see* Chapter 33).
Despite these trade-offs, reduced receive bandwidths should be used when a short TE is not required (T2 weighting) and when fat is not present. Examples are the brain, and in any examination when fat is suppressed.

29 Contrast-to-noise ratio (CNR)

The **contrast-to-noise ratio** or **CNR** is defined as the difference in SNR between two adjacent areas. It is controlled by the same factors that affect SNR. The CNR is probably the most important image quality factor, as the objective of any examination is to produce an image where pathology is clearly seen relative to normal anatomy. Visualization of a lesion increases if the CNR between it and surrounding anatomy is high. The CNR is increased by the administration of a contrast agent, magnetization transfer contrast, chemical suppression techniques and T2 weighting.

The administration of a contrast agent

Contrast agents such as gadolinium produce T1 shortening of lesions,

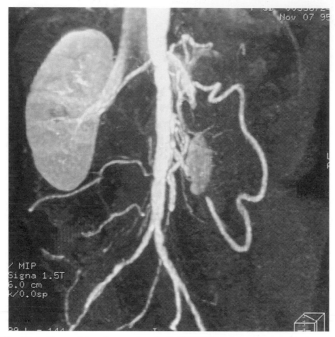

Fig. 29.1 Coronal incoherent (spoiled) GRE T1 weighted image during the first pass of contrast enhancement.

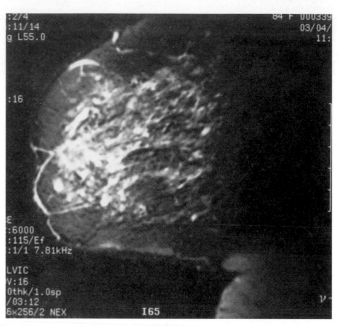

Fig. 29.2 Sagittal FSE T2 weighted image with chemical/spectral pre-saturation demonstrating high signal intensity throughout the breast.

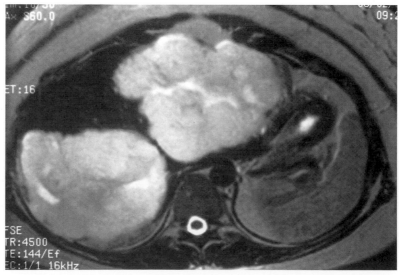

Fig. 29.3 Axial FSE T2 weighted image demonstrates a large mass as high signal intensity in the right and left lobes of the liver.

especially those that cause a breakdown in the blood–brain barrier. As a result, enhancing tissue appears bright on T1 weighted images (Fig. 29.1) and therefore there is a good CNR between it and surrounding non-enhancing tissue (see Chapter 42).

Magnetization transfer contrast (MTC)

MTC uses additional RF pulses to suppress hydrogen protons that are not free but bound to macromolecules and cell membranes. These pulses are either applied at a frequency away from the Larmor frequency where they are known as off resonant, or nearer to the centre frequency where they are known as on resonant. As a result of the application of these pulses, magnetization is transferred to the free protons, suppressing the signal in certain types of tissues.

Chemical suppression techniques

These can be used to suppress signal from either fat or water (Fig. 29.2). Fat suppression pulses are applied to the FOV prior to the excitation pulse resulting in nulling of fat signal. As a consequence, the CNR between lesions and surrounding normal tissues that contain fat is enhanced.

T2 weighting

T2 weighting is specifically used to increase the CNR between normal and abnormal tissue (Fig. 29.3). Pathology is often bright on a T2 weighted image as it contains water. As a result pathology is more conspicuous than on T1 or PD weighted images.

Sometimes acquiring an image with good CNR means compromising other image quality factors. An example is in the liver when, in T1 weighted images, lesions and normal liver may be **iso-intense** (the same signal intensity). By selecting fat suppressed T2 weighted imaging sequences, although SNR, spatial resolution and scan time are usually compromised because of the parameters selected, the CNR between lesions (bright) and normal liver (dark) is increased.

30 Spatial resolution

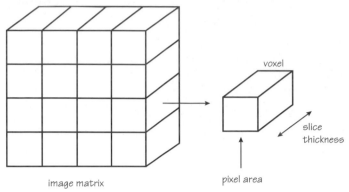

image matrix   pixel area

Fig. 30.1 The voxel.

Spatial resolution is defined as the ability to distinguish between two points that are close together in the patient. It is entirely controlled by the size of the **voxel**.
• The imaging volume is divided into **slices**.
• Each slice displays an area of anatomy defined as the **field of view (FOV)**.
• The FOV is divided into **pixels**, the size of which is controlled by **the matrix**. There are usually either 256 or 512 pixels along the frequency axis of the FOV and either 128, 192, 256, 384 or 512 pixels along the phase axis of the FOV.
• The phase matrix determines how many lines of K space are filled during data acquisition and therefore the scan time (see Chapters 25 and 26).
• The voxel is defined as the pixel area multiplied by the slice thickness. Therefore the factors that affect the **voxel volume** (Fig. 30.1) are:
  • slice thickness
  • FOV
  • the matrix.

Voxel volume and SNR
The size of the voxel determines how much signal each voxel contains. Large voxels have a higher signal than small ones because there are more spins in a large voxel to contribute to the signal. Therefore any setting of FOV, matrix size or slice thickness that results in large voxels leads to a higher SNR per voxel.

Voxel volume and spatial resolution
Small voxels improve resolution as they increase the likelihood of two points, close together in the patient, being in separate voxels and therefore distinguishable from each other. Changing any dimension of the voxel changes the resolution, but there is a direct trade-off with SNR.

Changing the matrix and SNR
Halving the matrix doubles the dimension of each pixel along the phase encoding axis. There are less pixels to map over a given FOV dimension in the phase direction, therefore each pixel is larger along this axis. The SNR of each voxel doubles.

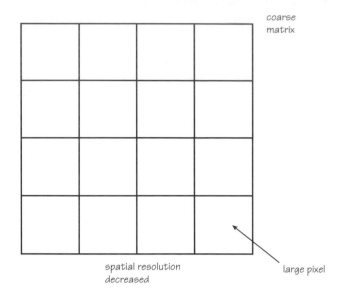

coarse matrix

spatial resolution decreased   large pixel

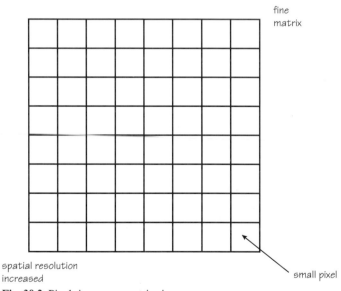

fine matrix

spatial resolution increased   small pixel

Fig. 30.2 Pixel size versus matrix size.

Changing the matrix and resolution
Changing the matrix alters the number of pixels that must fit into the FOV (Fig. 30.2). Therefore as the matrix increases, pixel, and therefore voxel size, decreases. As changing the phase matrix changes scan time, this factor is also affected.

The images in Fig. 30.3 were acquired with exactly the same parameters except that the right-hand image has a much finer matrix than the left-hand one. There are twice the number of frequency pixels and four times the number of phase pixels. As a result the resolution is increased but the SNR is reduced. In addition, as the phase matrix is four times higher, this image took four times longer to acquire.

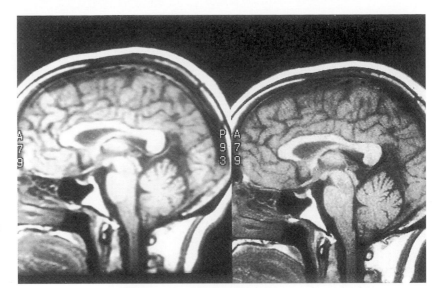

Fig. 30.3 Sagittal images of the brain. The image on the left was acquired with a matrix of 256×128, whereas the image on the right was acquired with a matrix of 512×256. The image on the right demonstrates improved spatial resolution. Which image took longer to acquire?

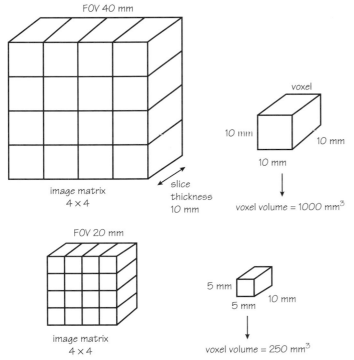

Fig. 30.4 FOV versus SNR.

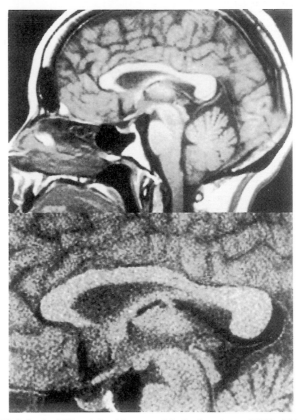

Fig. 30.5 Sagittal T1 weighted images of the brain using an FOV of 24 cm (above) and 12 cm (below). The lower image has greater spatial resolution, but a much reduced SNR.

Changing the FOV and SNR

When increasing the FOV pixel dimensions along each axis increase because the same number of pixels needs to cover a larger FOV, e.g. from a 12 cm FOV to a 24 cm FOV. The SNR of each voxel increases by a factor of four because the size of each pixel has doubled along each axis.

Changing the FOV and resolution

In Fig. 30.4 a FOV of 40 mm, a non-representative matrix of 4×4 and a slice of thickness 10 mm are illustrated. This produces a voxel volume of 1000 mm³. Halving the FOV to 20 mm reduces the voxel volume and therefore the SNR to a quarter of its original size, although spatial resolution is doubled along both the frequency and phase axes.

The images in Fig. 30.5 were acquired with exactly the same parameters, except the lower image has half the FOV of the top image. The lower image has better spatial resolution but lower SNR than the top image. As reducing the FOV affects the size of the pixel along both axes, the voxel volume is significantly reduced. Decreasing the FOV therefore has a drastic effect on SNR. Using a small FOV is appropriate when using small coils that boost local SNR but should be employed with caution when using a large coil as SNR will be severely compro-

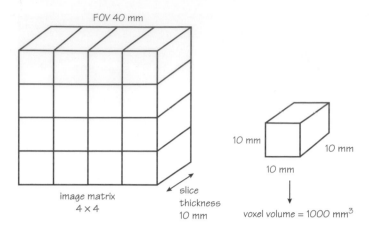

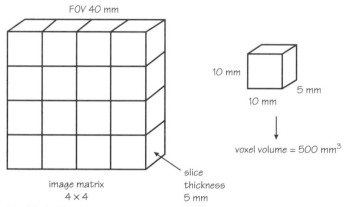

Fig. 30.6 Slice thickness versus SNR.

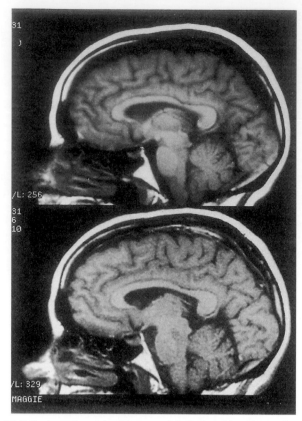

Fig. 30.7 Sagittal T1 weighted images of the brain with a 10 mm slice thickness (above) and a 3 mm slice thickness (below). The lower image has greater resolution but a lower SNR.

mised unless measures such as increasing the number of signal averages are taken.

Changing slice thickness and SNR

Increasing the slice thickness increases the voxel volume along the dimension of the slice. Thick slices cover more of the patient's body tissue and therefore have more spinning protons within them. SNR therefore increases in proportion to increase in slice thickness.

Changing slice thickness and resolution

In Fig. 30.6 a FOV of 40 mm, a non-representative matrix of 4×4 pixels and a slice thickness of 10 mm are illustrated. This produces a voxel volume of 1000 mm^3. Halving the slice thickness halves the voxel volume to 500 mm^3. As a result, spatial resolution is doubled in the plane of slice acquisition. However, as the voxel is now half the size of the original, the SNR is also halved as there are fewer spins in small voxels than in large ones.

The images in Fig. 30.7 were acquired with exactly the same parameters, except the top image has a slice thickness of 10 mm compared with the thickness in the lower image of 3 mm. The lower image has marginally better resolution but less SNR.

Sometimes however resolution can be increased without a corresponding increase in scan time. This can be done by changing the frequency matrix or using assymetric FOV.

Changing the frequency matrix only

The frequency matrix does not affect scan time, but if increased increases resolution. Therefore a higher resolution image can be acquired in the same time as a lower resolution image because only the phase matrix (which is unchanged) affects scan time.

Using asymmetric FOV

This maintains the size of the FOV along the frequency axis but reduces the FOV in the phase direction. Therefore the resolution of a square FOV is maintained but the scan time is reduced in proportion to the reduction in the size of the FOV in the phase direction. This option is useful when anatomy fits into a rectangle as in sagittal imaging of the pelvis. See Chapter 36 for K space filling and asymmetrical FOV.

31 Scan time

The scan time is determined by a combination of the TR, phase matrix and NEX:

$$\text{scan time} = \text{TR} \times \text{number of phase encodings} \times \text{NEX}$$

The longer a patient has to lie on the table, the more likely it is that he/she will move and ruin the image. Therefore it is important to reduce scan times and make the patient as comfortable as possible. Good immobilization is also essential as a couple of minutes spent doing this may save you many more minutes in wasted sequences. To reduce scan times either the TR and/or the phase matrix and/or the number of signal averages must be decreased. However there are trade-offs associated with this.

Reducing the TR:
• reduces the SNR because less longitudinal magnetization recovers during each TR period so that there is less to convert to transverse magnetization and therefore signal;
• reduces the number of slices available in a single acquisition as there is less time to excite and rephase slices, and
• increases T1 weighting because the tissues are more likely to be saturated.

Reducing the phase matrix:
• reduces resolution because there are fewer pixels in the phase axis of the image and therefore two areas close together in the patient are less likely to be spatially separated.

Reducing NEX/NSA:
• reduces SNR because data from the signal are sampled and stored in K space less often, and
• increases some motion artefact because averaging of noise is less.
  In two-dimensional sequences:

$$\text{scan time} = \text{TR} \times \text{number of phase encodings} \times \text{NEX}$$

In three-dimensional fast scan sequences:

$$\text{scan time} = \text{TR} \times \text{number of phase encodings} \times \text{NEX} \times \text{slice encodings}$$

Three-dimensional scans apply a second phase encoding gradient to select and excite each slice location so that scan time is also affected by the number of slice locations required in the volume.

Table 32.1 The results of optimizing image quality.

To optimize image	Adjusted parameter	consequence
Maximize SNR	↑ NEX	↑ scan time
	↓ matrix	↓ scan time
		↓ spatial resolution
	↑ slice thickness	↓ spatial resolution
	↓ receive bandwidth	↑ minimum TE
		↑ chemical shift
	↑ FOV	↓ spatial resolution
	↑ TR	↓ T1 weighting
		↑ number of slices
	↓ TE	↓ T2 weighting
Maximize spatial resolution (assuming a square FOV)	↓ slice thickness	↓ SNR
	↑ matrix	↓ SNR
		↑ scan time
	↓ FOV	↓ SNR
Minimize scan time		↑ T1 weighting
	↓ TR	↓ SNR
		↓ number of slices
	↓ phase encodings	↓ spatial resolution
		↑ SNR
	↓ NEX	↑ SNR
		↑ movement artefact
	↓ slice number in volume imaging	↓ SNR

Table 32.2 Parameters and their associated trade-offs.

Parameter	Benefit	Limitation
TR increased	increased SNR increased number of slices	increased scan time decreased T1 weighting
TR decreased	decreased scan time increased T1 weighting	decreased SNR decreased number of slices
TE increased	increased T2 weighting	decreased SNR
TE decreased	increased SNR	decreased T2 weighting
NEX increased	increased SNR more signal averaging	direct proportional increase in scan time
NEX decreased	direct proportional decrease in scan time	decreased SNR less signal averaging
Slice thickness increased	increased SNR increased coverage of anatomy	decreased spatial resolution more partial voluming
Slice thickness decreased	increased spatial resolution reduced partial voluming	decreased SNR decreased coverage of anatomy
FOV increased	increased SNR increased coverage of anatomy	decreased spatial resolution decreased likelihood of aliasing
FOV decreased	increased spatial resolution increased likelihood of aliasing	decreased SNR decreased coverage of anatomy
Matrix incresed	increased spatial resolution	increased scan time decreased SNR if pixel is small
Matrix decreased	decreased scan time increased SNR if pixel is large	decreased spatial resolution
Receive bandwidth increased	decrease in chemical shift decrease in minimum TE	decreased SNR
Receive bandwidth decreased	increased SNR	increase in chemical shift increase in minimum TE
Large coil	increased area of received signal	lower SNR sensitive to artefacts aliasing with small FOV
Small coil	increased SNR less sensitive to artefacts less prone to aliasing with a small FOV	decreased area of received signal

33 Chemical shift

Mechanism

Chemical shift artefact is a displacement of signal between fat and water along the frequency axis of the image. It is caused by the dissimilar chemical environments of fat and water that produces a precessional frequency difference between the magnetic moments of fat and water. In water, hydrogen is linked to oxygen; in fat it is linked to carbon. Because of the two different chemical environments, hydrogen in fat resonates at a lower frequency than water. There is therefore a **frequency shift** inherently present between fat and water. Its magnitude depends on the magnetic field strength of the system and significantly increases at higher field strengths.

The **receive bandwidth** is one of the factors that controls chemical

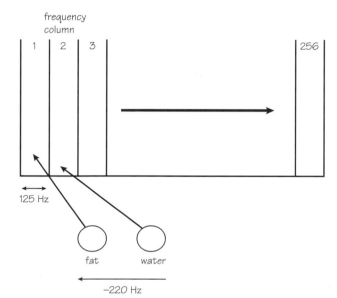

Fig. 33.1 Chemical shift at 1.5 T.

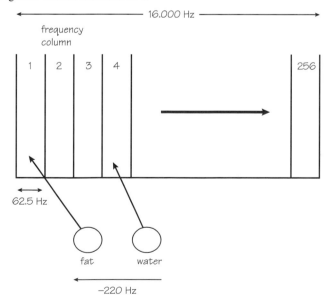

Fig. 33.2 Chemical shift at reduced bandwidth.

shift. It also controls SNR (see Chapter 28). The receive bandwidth determines the range of frequencies that must be mapped across either 512 or 256 pixels in the frequency direction of the FOV. It is selected to receive signal with frequencies slightly higher and lower than the centre frequency. It is usually measured in KHz (kilo hertz). At 1.5 T with a receive bandwidth of +/−16 KHz on each side of the centre frequency, each pixel contains a range of frequencies of either 125 Hz or 62.5 Hz, depending on the frequency matrix (Fig. 33.1). Where fat and water co-exist in the patient, the frequency encoding process maps fat hydrogen several Hz lower than water hydrogen. They therefore appear in different pixels in the image despite co-existing in the patient. As the receive bandwidth is reduced, fewer frequencies are mapped across the same number of pixels. As a result chemical shift artefact increases (Fig. 33.2).

Appearance

Chemical shift artefact causes a signal void between areas of fat and water. An example is around the kidneys where the water-filled kidneys are surrounded by peri-renal fat (Fig. 33.3).

Remedies

- Scan with a low field strength magnet.
- Remove either the fat or water signal by the use of STIR/chemical/spectral pre-saturation.
- Broaden the receive bandwidth (what is the trade-off?).

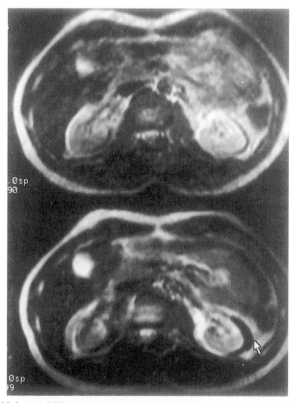

Fig. 33.3 Axial T2 weighted images of the abdomen using a receive bandwidth of 32 000 Hz (above), and 8000 Hz (below). The arrow demonstrates chemical shift artefact at the border of the left kidney.

34 Chemical misregistration

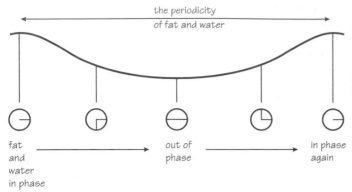

Fig. 34.1 The periodicity of fat and water.

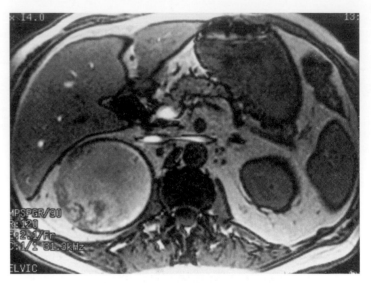

Fig. 34.2 Axial incoherent (spoiled) GRE T1 weighted image acquired with a TE when fat and water are out of phase.

Mechanism

Chemical misregistration is caused by the difference in precessional frequency between fat and water that results in their magnetic moments being in phase with each other at certain times and out of phase at others. When the signals from both fat and water are out of phase, they cancel each other out so that signal loss results (Fig. 34.1). If an image is produced when fat and water are out of phase, an artefact called **chemical misregistration** results. The time interval between fat and water being in phase is called the **periodicity**. This time depends on the frequency shift and therefore the field strength. At 1.5 T the periodicity is 4.2 ms. At lower field strengths the periodicity of fat and water is shorter.

Appearance

An out of phase image produces an asymmetrical edging effect in the phase direction. This artefact mainly occurs along the phase axis and causes a dark ring around structures that contain both fat and water (Fig. 34.2). It is most prevalent in gradient echo sequences because gradient rephasing cannot compensate for the phase difference as well as RF rephasing.

Remedies

• Use SE or FSE/TSE pulse sequences (which use RF rephasing pulses).
• Use a TE that matches the periodicity of fat and water so that the echo is generated when fat and water are in phase.
• **The Dixon technique** involves selecting a TE at half the periodicity so that fat and water are out of phase. In this way the signal from fat is reduced. This technique is mainly effective in areas where water and fat co-exist in a voxel.

35 Magnetic susceptibility

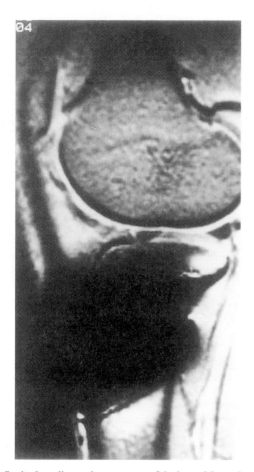

Fig. 35.1 Sagittal gradient echo sequence of the knee. Magnetic susceptibility artefact from the screws degrades the image.

Mechanism

Magnetic susceptibility artefact occurs because all tissues magnetize to a different degree depending on their magnetic characteristics (see Chapter 1). This produces a difference in their individual precessional frequencies and phase. The phase discrepancy causes dephasing at the boundaries of structures with a very different magnetic susceptibility, and signal loss results

Appearance

Areas of signal void and high signal intensity often accompanied by distortion are produced. It is commonly seen on gradient echo sequences when the patient has a metal prosthesis in situ (Fig. 35.1) but is also visualized at the interface of the petrous bone and the brain. Magnetic susceptibility can be used advantageously when investigating haemorrhage or blood products, as the presence of this artefact suggests that bleeding has recently occurred (Fig. 35.2).

Remedies

- Use SE or FSE pulse sequences that use RF rephasing pulses.
- Removing all metal items from the patient before the examination.

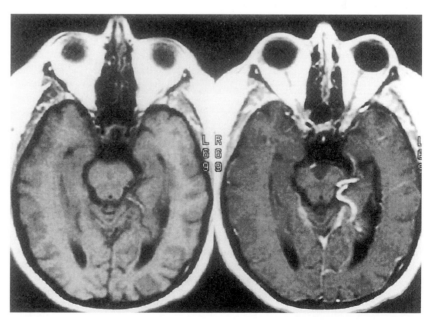

Fig. 35.2 These axial images of the brain were acquired to evaluate the arterio-venous malformation (AVM) in the posterior parietal lobe of the brain. The T2 fast spin echo (left) demonstrates subtle findings whereas the T2* gradient echo (right) shows a large susceptibility artefact in the same area caused by blood.

36 Phase mismapping (motion artefact)

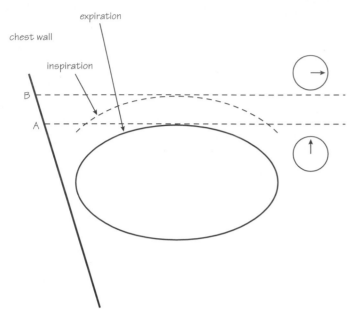

Fig. 36.1 How ghosting occurs.

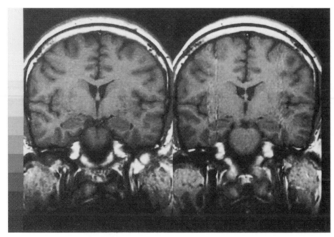

Fig. 36.2 Coronal FSE T1 weighted images through the temporal lobes. The image on the left has the phase encoding axis R to L. The image on the right has the phase encoding axis S to I. Artefact is removed from the lateral portion of the temporal lobes on this image but interferes with the hippocampal region.

Mechanism

Phase artefact results from anatomy moving between the application of the phase encoding gradient and the frequency encoding gradient (intra-view) and motion between each application of the phase gradient (view to view). If anatomy moves during these periods it is assigned the wrong phase value and is mismapped onto the image. It causes an artefact called **ghosting** or **phase mismapping** and always occurs along the phase axis of the image.

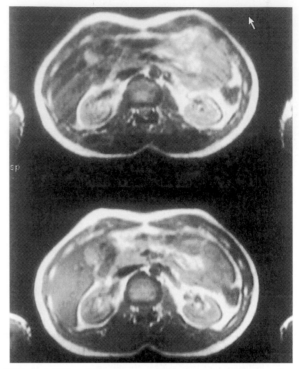

Fig. 36.3 Axial T1 weighted images of the abdomen without respiratory compensation (above), and using respiratory compensation (below). The ghosting (arrow), has been reduced on the lower image.

In Fig. 36.1 the abdominal wall is at one position when the phase encoding gradient is applied, and a phase shift value is allocated to it according to its position on the phase encoding gradient. If the abdominal wall has moved to another position during readout, the system still allocates a location along the phase axis according to the first position. The most common causes of phase mismapping are respiration, which moves the chest and abdominal wall along the phase encoding gradient, and pulsatile movement of artery or venous walls.

Appearance

There is blurring or ghosting across the image.

Remedies

Swapping the phase and frequency direction removes the artefact from the area of interest. Note this does not eliminate it; it only moves it away from the area of interest (Fig. 36.2).

Using respiratory compensation reduces phase mismapping from the motion of the chest wall along the phase encoding gradient during the acquisition of data (Fig. 36.3). This is achieved by placing expandable air filled bellows around the patient's chest. The movement of air back

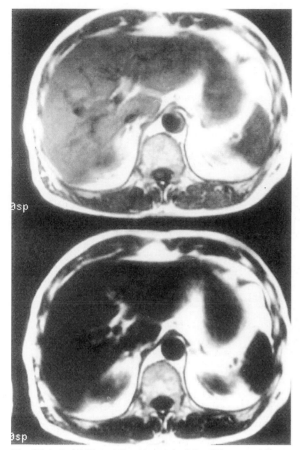

Fig. 36.4 Axial T1 weighted images of the abdomen without water pre-saturation (above), and with water pre-saturation (below). Note how the signal intensity is reduced in the liver on the lower image.

and forth along the bellows during inspiration and expiration, is converted to a waveform by a transducer. The system then orders the phase encoding gradients so that the steep slopes occur when maximum movement of the chest wall occurs, and reserves the shallow gradient slopes for minimum chest wall motion. In this way most of the signal is acquired when the chest wall is relatively still and therefore phase ghosting is reduced.

Pre-saturation delivers a 90° RF pulse to a volume of tissue outside the FOV. This is called a **saturation band**. A flowing nucleus within the volume receives this 90° pulse. When it enters the slice stack, it receives an excitation pulse and is saturated. If it is fully saturated to 180°, it has no transverse component of magnetization and produces a signal void. To be effective, pre-saturation pulses should be placed between the flow and the imaging stack so that signal from flowing nuclei entering the FOV is nullified. Spatial saturation increases the rate of RF delivery to the patient, this increases the SAR.

Chemical presaturation is used to produce a signal void in either fat or water. Hydrogen nuclei exist in two different chemical environments: the precessional frequencies of hydrogen in each environment are different. This precessional frequency shift is called **chemical shift**

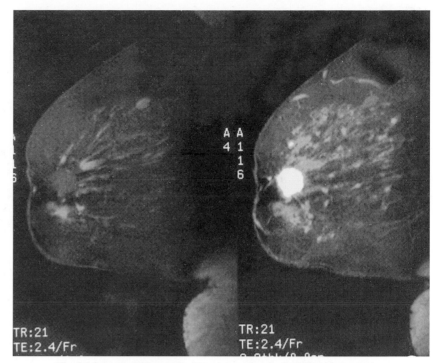

Fig. 36.5 Sagittal T1 weighted incoherent (spoiled) GRE with spectral pre-saturation before (left) and after (right) contrast enhancement.

because it is caused by a difference in the chemical environments of fat and water. Chemical shift causes artefacts but also provides an opportunity to use a presaturation pulse to eliminate signal from either water or fat. This is called **chemical presaturation**.

Water sat
The chemical saturation RF pulse applied at the precessional frequency of water hydrogen shifts the NMV of water into saturation. The water hydrogen therefore has no transverse magnetization and thus no signal. When the signal from water is suppressed this is called water suppression (Fig. 36.4).

Fat sat
The chemical saturation RF pulse is transmitted at the precessional frequency of fat hydrogen to shift the NMV of fat hydrogen into saturation. The fat hydrogen nuclei have no magnetization in the transverse plane and thus no signal. The fat signal is now suppressed (Fig. 36.5).

Gradient moment rephasing (nulling/flow compensation) for the altered phase values of the nuclei flowing along a gradient see Chapter 38. It uses additional gradients to correct the altered phases back to their original values. In this way, flowing nuclei do not gain or lose phase due to the presence of the main gradient. Gradient moment rephasing therefore gives flowing nuclei a bright signal as they are in phase. As gradient moment rephasing uses extra gradients, it increases the minimum TE.

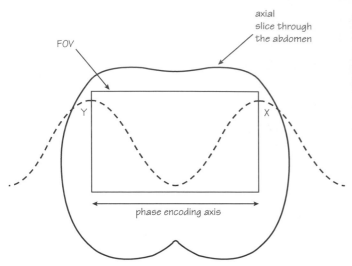

Fig. 37.1 X and Y have the same value of phase.

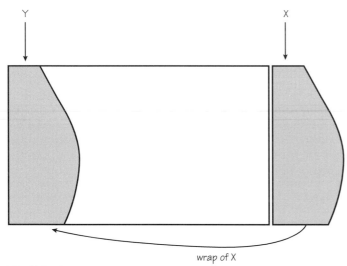

Fig. 37.2 Phase wrap.

Mechanism

This occurs when anatomy that is producing signal exists outside the FOV in the phase direction. Within the FOV, a finite number of phase values from 0° to 360° must be mapped into the FOV in the phase direction. This can be represented as a 'phase curve' that is repeated on either side of the FOV in the phase direction. Owing to the finite number of phase values, signal coming from X has the same phase value as signal coming from Y because they are both in the same position on the phase curve (Fig. 37.1). There is therefore a duplication of phase values for anatomy inside and outside the FOV (undersampling).

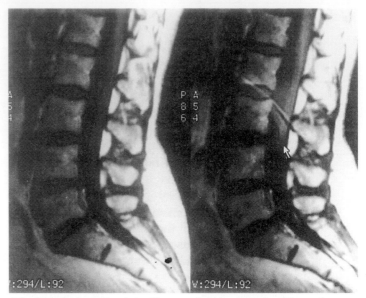

Fig. 37.3 Sagittal T1 weighted images of the lumbar spine. The artefact (arrow) is phase wrap. The image on the left was acquired using anti-aliasing measures.

Appearance

Anatomy at position X is mapped onto the image at position Y. This is called **wrap around**, **fold-over** or **aliasing** (Fig. 37.2). Anatomy from one side of the image overlaps the other (Fig. 37.3). Severe forms can ruin an image.

Remedies

Aliasing can occur along the frequency axis but is usually automatically compensated for. Phase wrap is reduced or eliminated in the following ways:
• by increasing the FOV to the boundaries of the coil;
• by placing spatial pre-saturation pulses over signal-producing anatomy;
• by **oversampling** in the phase direction. This is specifically called **anti-aliasing**. During data acquisition the FOV is doubled in the phase direction so that the phase curve now extends over twice the distance of the original FOV. There is now no duplication of phase shift values of signal from anatomy outside the FOV. The matrix is doubled to compensate for the reduced spatial resolution as a result of doubling the FOV. The NEX/NSA are usually halved to compensate for doubling the phase matrix. During image reconstruction the extra FOV is discarded (only the middle portion corresponding to the FOV selected is displayed). There is usually no penalty in scan time, signal or spatial resolution when using anti-aliasing, although motion artefact may be increased due to less signal averaging. See Chapter 27 for K space filling and anti-aliasing.

38 Flow phenomena

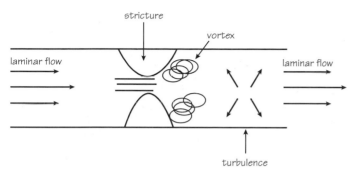

Fig. 38.1 The different types of flow.

Laminar flow is flow that is at different but consistent velocities across a vessel. The flow at the centre of the lumen of the vessel is faster than at the vessel wall, where resistance slows down the flow. However, the velocity difference across the vessel is constant (Fig. 38.1).

Turbulent flow is flow at different velocities that fluctuates randomly. The velocity difference across the vessel changes erratically.

Vortex flow is flow that is initially laminar but then passes through a stricture or stenosis in the vessel. Flow in the centre of the lumen has a high velocity but, near the walls, the flow spirals.

Stagnant flow is where the velocity of flow slows to a point of stagnation. The signal intensity of stagnant flow depends on its T1, T2 and proton density characteristics. It behaves like stationary tissue.

Flow mechanisms are often termed as follows:

First order motion	laminar flow
Second order motion	acceleration
Third order motion	jerk

Only first order flow can be compensated for.

Time of flight phenomenon

In order to produce a signal, a nucleus must receive an excitation pulse and a rephasing pulse. Stationary nuclei always receive both excitation and rephasing pulses. Flowing nuclei present in the slice for the excitation may have exited the slice before rephasing. This is called **time of flight phenomenon** (Fig. 38.2). If a nucleus receives the excitation pulse only and is not rephased, it does not produce a signal. If a nucleus is rephased but has not previously been excited, it does not produce a signal. Time of flight effects depend on:
• the velocity of flow;
• the TE;
• the slice thickness.

Flow related enhancement increases as:
• the velocity of flow decreases;

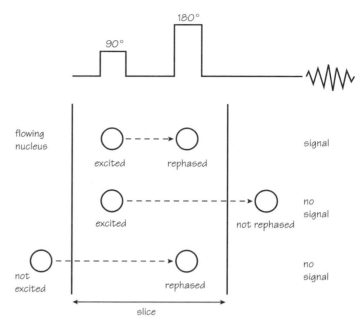

Fig. 38.2 The time of flight phenomenon.

• the TE decreases;
• the slice thickness increases.
High velocity signal void increases as:
• the velocity of flow increases;
• the TE increases;
• the slice thickness decreases.

Entry slice phenomenon (in-flow effect)

The **entry slice phenomenon** is related to the excitation history of the nuclei. Nuclei that receive repeated RF pulses during the acquisition are saturated. Nuclei that have not received these repeated RF pulses are 'fresh', as their magnetic moments have not been saturated by successive RF pulses. The signal that they produce is different from that of the saturated nuclei.

Stationary nuclei within a slice become saturated after repeated RF pulses. Nuclei flowing perpendicular to the slice enter the slice fresh, as they were not present during repeated excitations. They therefore produce a different signal from the stationary nuclei. This is called the **entry slice phenomenon** as it is most prominent in the first and last slices of a 'stack' of slices. The slices in the middle of the stack exhibit less entry slice phenomenon, as flowing nuclei have received more excitation pulses by the time they reach these slices.

Any factor that affects the rate at which a nucleus receives repeated excitations affects the magnitude of the phenomenon. The magnitude of entry slice phenomenon therefore depends on:

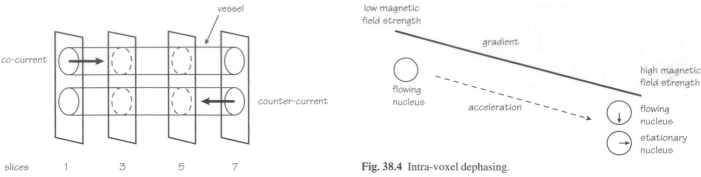

Fig. 38.3 Co- and counter-current flow.

Fig. 38.4 Intra-voxel dephasing.

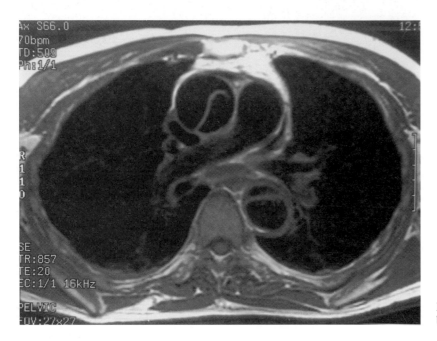

Fig. 38.5 Axial T1 weighted SE image of the chest using black blood imaging.

- the TR;
- the slice thickness;
- the velocity of flow;
- the direction of flow.

Direction of flow

Co-current flow Flow that is in the **same** direction as slice selection is called **co-current**. The flowing nuclei are more likely to receive repeated RF excitations as they move from one slice to the next. They therefore become saturated relatively quickly, and so entry slice phenomenon decreases rapidly (Fig. 38.3).

Counter current flow Flow that is in the **opposite** direction to slice selection is called **counter-current** flow. Flowing nuclei stay fresh as when they enter a slice they are less likely to have received previous excitation pulses. Entry slice phenomenon does not therefore decrease rapidly and may still be present deep within the slice stack (Fig. 38.3).

Intra-voxel dephasing

Nuclei flowing along a gradient rapidly accelerate or decelerate depending on the direction of flow and gradient application. Flowing nuclei either gain phase (if they have been accelerated), or lose phase (if they have been decelerated). If a flowing nucleus is adjacent to a stationary nucleus in a voxel, there is a phase difference between the two nuclei. This is because the flowing nucleus has either lost or gained phase relative to the stationary nucleus due to its motion along the gradient. Nuclei within the same voxel are out of phase with each other, which results in a reduction of total signal amplitude from the voxel. This is called **intra-voxel dephasing** (Fig. 38.4).

Black blood imaging (Fig. 38.5)

This technique uses conventional T1 weighted spin echo sequences with pre-saturation pulses, to visualize flowing vessels that appear black in contrast to surrounding structures. Saturation eliminates phase ghosting and provides intra-luminal signal void to distinguish between patent and obstructed vessels. It can be used to evaluate vascular patency especially in the neck, brain, chest and abdomen. As flowing blood appears black, persistent signal within vessel lumen after the application of saturation pulses indicates either stagnant flow within the vessel, or vascular occlusion.

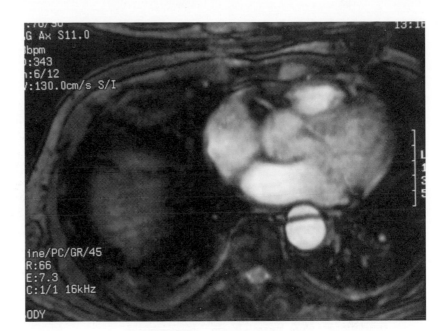

Fig. 38.6 Axial coherent GRE T2* cine image of the heart and great vessels using bright blood imaging. Note the high signal intensity in the vessels and the flap in the descending aorta indicating a dissection.

Bright blood imaging (Fig. 38.6)

This technique uses gradient moment nulling, usually in conjunction with coherent gradient echo sequences, to make flowing blood bright. Gradient moment rephasing complements flow by making vessels containing slow flowing spins appear bright, so enhancing the signal from blood and CSF. Gradient moment rephasing is widely used in the chest and abdomen, brain, extremities and for the myelographic effect of CSF in T2 weighted images of the spine. As GMN requires a longer minimum TE due to the use of additional gradients, a reduction in the number of slices available often results.

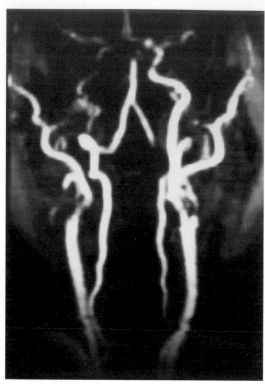

Fig. 39.1 Coronal triggered 2D TOF-MRA through the carotids and bifurcation.

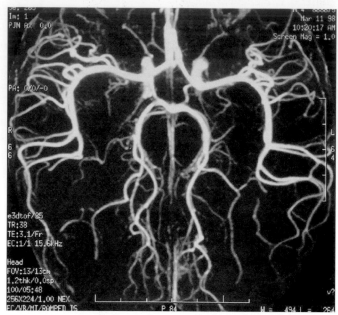

Fig. 39.2 3D TOF-MRA in a 4-year-old child showing normal appearances.

Mechanism

Time of flight MRA (TOF-MRA) produces vascular contrast by manipulating longitudinal magnetization of stationary spins. It uses a gradient echo pulse sequence in combination with GMN to enhance signal in flowing vessels. The TR is kept well below the T1 time of the stationary tissues so that T1 recovery is prevented. This saturates the stationary spins, whilst the in-flow effect from fully magnetized flowing fresh spins produces high vascular signal. However if the TR is too short, the flowing spins may be suppressed along with the stationary spins that reduce vascular contrast. To evaluate signals from arterial flow, saturation pulses are applied in the direction of venous flow. For example, to evaluate the carotid arteries in the neck, apply saturation pulses superior to the imaging volume to saturate the signal from inflowing venous blood (Fig. 39.1). TOF-MRA is only sensitive to flow that comes into the FOV. Any flow that traverses the FOV can be saturated along with the stationary tissue.

2D vs. 3D TOF-MRA

TOF-MRA is acquired in either 2D (slice by slice) or 3D (volume) acquisition modes. In general, 3D volume imaging offers high SNR and thin contiguous slices for good resolution (Fig. 39.2). However, as TOF-MRA is sensitive to flow coming into the FOV or the imaging volume, spins in vessels with slow flow can be saturated in volume imaging. For this reason, 3D TOF should be used in areas of high velocity flow (intra-cranial applications) and 2D TOF in areas of slower velocity flow (carotids, peripheral vascular and the venous systems). In 3D techniques, there is a higher risk of saturating signals from spins within the volume.

Clinical uses

The carotid bifurcation, the peripheral circulation and cortical venous mapping can be imaged with 2D TOF-MRA.

Parameters

- TR 45 ms
- Minimum allowable TE
- Flip angles approximately 60°
- The TR and flip angle saturate stationary nuclei but moving spins coming into the slice remain fresh, so image contrast is maximized.
- The short TE reduces phase ghosting.
- Gradient moment rephasing, in conjunction with saturation pulses to suppress signals from areas of undesired flow, are used to enhance vascular contrast.

General TOF advantages

- Sensitive to T1 effects (short T1 tissues are bright. Contrast may be given for additional enhancement).

- Reasonable imaging times (approximately 5 min depending on parameters).
- Sensitive to slow flow.
- Reduced sensitivity to intra-voxel dephasing.

General TOF disadvantages

- Sensitive to T1 effects (short T1 tissues are bright so that hemorrhagic lesions may mimic vessels).
- Saturation of in-plane flow (any flow within the FOV or volume of tissue can be saturated along with background tissue).
- Enhancement is limited to either flow entering the FOV or very high velocity flow.

Table 39.1 2D *vs.* 3D time of flight.

2D TOF advantages	2D TOF disadvantages
Large area of coverage	lower resolution
Sensitive to slow flow	saturation of in-plane flow
Sensitive to T1 effects	Venetian blind artefact
3D TOF advantages	**3D TOF disadvantages**
High resolution for small vessels	saturation of in-plane flow
Sensitive to T1 effects	small area of coverage

Table 39.2 Overcoming disadvantages of TOF-MRA.

Susceptibility artefacts	Use short TEs and small voxel volumes.
Poor background suppression	Use TEs that acquire data when fat and water are out of phase.
	Implement magnetization transfer techniques.
Venetian blind artefacts	Use breath-hold techniques.
Limited coverage (3D)	Acquire images in another plane.
	Use MOTSA (multiple overlapping thin section angiography).
Suppression of in-plane signal	Use ramped RF pulses.
	Administer contrast media.
Pulsation artefacts	Time acquisition to the cardiac cycle.

40 Phase contrast MRA (PC-MRA)

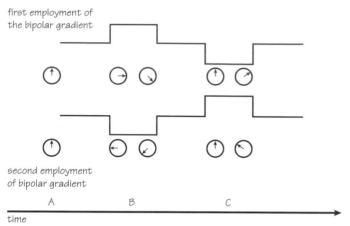

Fig. 40.1 Bipolar gradients to produce phase contrast.

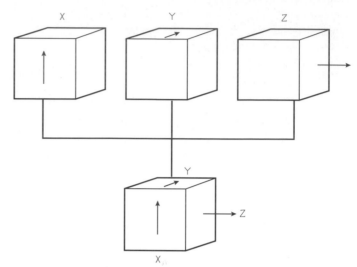

Fig. 40.2 Flow encoding axes.

Mechanism

Phase contrast MRA utilizes velocity changes, and hence phase shifts in moving spins, to provide image contrast in flowing vessels. Phase shifts are generated in the pulse sequence by phase encoding the velocity of flow with the use of a bipolar (two lobes, one negative one positive) gradient. Phase shift is introduced selectively for moving spins with the use of magnetic field gradients. This technique is known as **phase contrast magnetic resonance angiography (PC-MRA)**. PC-MRA is sensitive to flow within, as well as that coming into the FOV.

- Immediately after the RF excitation pulse spins are in phase (time *A*) (Fig. 40.1), a gradient is applied to both stationary and flowing spins. Although phase shifts occur in both stationary and flowing spins, these shifts occur at different rates.
- During initial application of the first bipolar gradient (time *B*), there is a shift of phases of stationary spins (left) and flowing spins (right).
- After the second part of the application of the first bipolar gradient (time *C*), the stationary spins (left) return to their initial phase (time *A*), but those of moving spins (right) acquire some phase.
- The bipolar gradient is then applied with opposite polarity so that the same variants occur, but in the opposite direction.
- PC-MRA then subtracts the two acquisitions so that the signals from stationary spins are subtracted out leaving only the signals from flowing spins. The combination of PC-MRA acquisitions results in what are known as magnitude and phase images.
- The unsubtracted combinations of flow sensitized image data are known as **magnitude** images.
- The subtracted combinations are called **phase** images.

The bipolar gradients induce phase shifts along their axes. By applying bipolar gradients in all three axes the sequence is sensitized to flow in all three directions X, Y and Z. These are known as **flow encoding axes** (Fig. 40.2). The sequence is also sensitized to flow velocity using a **velocity encoding technique (VENC)** that compensates for projected flow velocity within vessels by controlling the amplitude or strength of the bipolar gradient. If the VENC selected is lower than the velocity within the vessel, aliasing can occur. This results in low signal intensity in the centre of the vessel, but better delineation of vessel wall itself. With high VENC settings, intra-luminal signal is improved, but vessel wall delineation is compromised.

2D vs. 3D PC-MRA

2D techniques provide acceptable imaging times and flow direction information. 2D acquisitions, however, cannot be reformatted and viewed in other imaging planes. 3D offers SNR and spatial resolution superior to 2D imaging strategies, and the ability to reformat in a number of imaging planes retrospectively. The trade-off however is that in 3D PC-MRA, imaging time increases with the TR, NEX, the number of phase encoding steps, the number of slices and the number of flow encoding axes selected. For this reason, scan times are sometimes long.

Clinical uses

PC-MRA can be used effectively in the evaluation of arteriovenous malformations, aneurysms, venous occlusions, congenital abnormalities and traumatic intra-cranial vascular injuries (Fig. 40.3).

Parameters
3D volume acquisitions

- 28 slices volume, 1 mm slice thickness
- Flip angle 20° (60 slice volume flip angle reduced to 15°)
- TR less than or equal to 25 ms
- VENC 40–60 cm/s
- Flow encoding in all directions

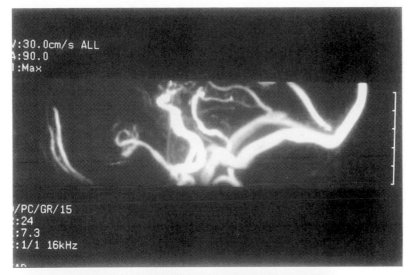

Fig. 40.3(a) This axial image of the brain was acquired with a 3D PC-MRA and projected in the sagittal plane. Parameters were chosen to visualize the venous flow in the transverse sinus as well as arterial flow up to the circle of Willis. Note that the background suppression is better than with TOF-MRA.

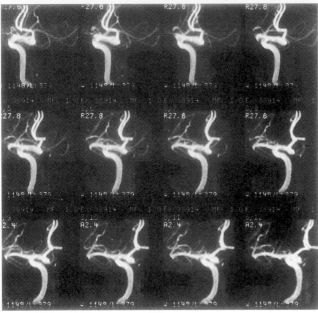

Fig. 40.3(b) This series of images represents post-processing for MRA whereby the vessel of interest is segmented out from the other vessels and projected in a number of obliquities. Note that the smaller vessels are visualized with depth on this MIP display as nearer vessels appear bright and vessels at the back appear dark.

2D techniques acquisitions

Cranial
- TR 18–20 ms
- Flip angle 20°
- Slices thickness 20–60 mm
- VENCs   20–30 cm/s for venous flow
          40–60 cm/s for higher velocity with some aliasing
          60–80 cm/s to determine velocity and flow direction

Carotid
- Flip angles 20° to 30°
- TR 20 ms
- VENCs   40–60 cm/s for better morphology with aliasing
          60–80 cm/s for quantitative velocity and directional information

Table 40.1 Phase contrast advantages and disadvantages.

Advantages of PC-MRA	Disadvantages of PC-MRA
Sensitivity to a variety of vascular velocities	long imaging times with 3D more sensitive to turbulence
Sensitivity to flow within the FOV	
Reduced intra-voxel dephasing	
Increased background suppression	
Magnitude and phase images	

41 Contrast enhanced MRA

Contrast mechanism

Gadolinium is a T1 shortening agent that enhances blood if given in sufficient quantities into the bloodstream. If used in conjunction with a T1 weighted sequence, blood appears bright and is well seen in contrast to surrounding non-enhancing tissues (see Chapter 42). A conventional or fast incoherent gradient echo sequence should therefore be used.

Administration

This is administered intravenously, usually via the ante-cubital fossa by hand or mechanical injection.

Doses must be sufficiently high to give adequate vessel delineation. 40 to 60 ml (about 0.3 mmol/kg) of gadolinium is required.

Image timing

To obtain an arterial-phase image in which arteries are bright and veins are dark, it is essential that the central K space data (i.e., the low spatial frequency data) are acquired while gadolinium concentration in the arteries is high but relatively lower in the veins (Figs 41.1 and 41.2).

The time it takes contrast to travel from the ante-cubital fossa to the area of interest depends on:
- the distance of the area from the injection site;
- the type of vessel (e.g. artery or vein);
- the velocity of flow;
- the speed of injection;
- the length of the acquisition.

For long acquisitions lasting more than 100 s, use sequential ordering of K space, so that the centre of K space is collected during the middle of the acquisition. Sequential ordering results in fewer artefacts. Begin injecting the gadolinium just after initiating imaging. Finish the injection just after the midpoint of the acquisition, being careful to maintain the maximum injection rate for the approximately 10–30 s prior to the middle of the acquisition. This will ensure a maximum arterial gadolinium during the middle of the acquisition when central K-space data are collected.

For short acquisitions less than 45 s contrast agent bolus timing is more critical and challenging. There are several approaches to determining the optimal bolus timing for these fast scans. For a typical breath-hold scan duration of 35–45 s in a reasonably healthy patient with an IV site in the ante-cubital vein, a delay of approximately 10–12 s is appropriate. Therefore, begin the injection, and then 10 s later start imaging while the patient suspends breathing.

More reliable and precise techniques are also available. These include:
- using a test bolus to measure the contrast travel time precisely;
- using an automatic pulse sequence that monitors signal in the aorta and then initiates imaging after contrast is detected arriving in the aorta;
- imaging so rapidly that bolus timing is unimportant.

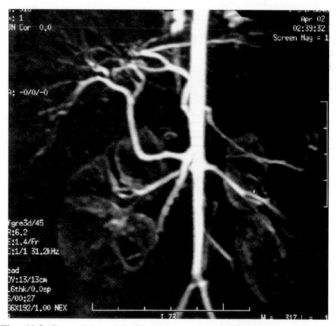

Fig. 41.2 Coronal breath-hold contrast-enhanced MRA using an incoherent (spoiled) GRE sequence in a 4-month-old child pre-liver transplant.

Table 41.1 Advantages and disadvantages of CE-MRA.

Advantages CE-MRA	Disadvantages CE-MRA
Easier to visualize vessels – fewer false positives.	Timing is sometimes difficult.
No extra sequences are needed.	It is invasive – there is risk of reaction.
With practice, examination complete in 15–30 mins.	Extra equipment such as power injectors and moving tables may be required.

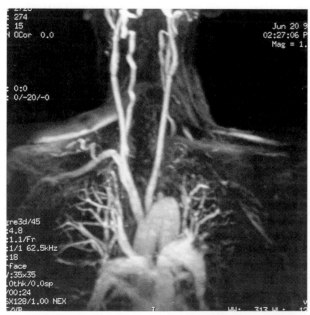

Fig. 41.1 Coronal contrast enhanced MRA of the great vessels and neck.

42 Contrast media

Mechanism of action

In order to increase contrast between pathology and normal tissue, enhancement agents may be introduced that selectively affect the T1 and T2 relaxation times in tissues. Both T1 recovery and T2 decay are influenced by the magnetic field experienced locally within the nucleus. The local magnetic field responsible for these processes is caused by:

• the main magnetic field;
• the fluctuations caused by the magnetic moments of nuclear spins in neighbouring molecules.

These molecules rotate or tumble, and the rate of rotation of the molecules is a characteristic property of the solution (Fig. 42.1). It is dependent on:

• the magnetic field strength;
• the viscosity of the solution;
• the temperature of the solution.

Molecules that tumble with a frequency at or near the Larmor frequency have more efficient T1 recovery times than other molecules.

Dipole–dipole interactions

The phenomenon by which excited protons are affected by nearby excited protons and electrons is called **dipole–dipole** interaction. If a tumbling molecule with a large magnetic moment such as gadolinium is placed in the presence of water protons, local magnetic field fluctuations occur near the Larmor frequency. T1 relaxation times of nearby protons are therefore reduced and so they appear bright on a T1 weighted image. This effect on a substance whereby relaxation rates are altered is known as **relaxivity**.

Gadolinium

Gadolinium (Gd) is a **paramagnetic** agent. It is a trivalent lanthanide element that has seven unpaired electrons and an ability to allow rapid exchange of bulk water to minimize the space between itself and water within the body. It has a large magnetic moment and when it is placed in the presence of tumbling water protons, fluctuations in the local magnetic field are created near the Larmor frequency. The T1 relaxation times of nearby water protons are therefore reduced, resulting in an increased signal intensity on T1 weighted images. For this reason, gadolinium is known as a **T1 enhancement agent**.

Chelation

Gadolinium is a rare-earth metal that cannot be excreted by the body and would cause long term side effects, as it binds to membranes. By binding the rare-earth metal ion gadolinium, with a **chelate** such as dienthylene triaminepentaacetic acid (DTPA) (a ligand), Gd-DTPA is formed which can be safely excreted. Other chelates include:

• HP-DO3A in which the charges have been balanced to produce a non-ionic contrast agent;
• DTPA-BMA (gadodiamide) a non-ionic linear molecule;
• Gd DOTA an ionic macrocyclic molecule (Fig. 42.2).

Side effects

• A slight transitory increase in bilirubin and blood iron
• Mild transitory headaches
• Nausea
• Vomiting
• Hypotension

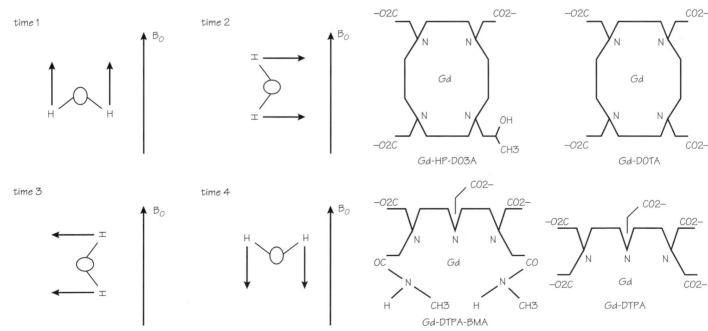

Fig. 42.1 Tumbling of water molecules.

Fig. 42.2 Molecular structures of gadolinium chelates.

- Gastro-intestinal upset
- Rash

Contra-indications
- Haematological disorders such as haemolytic anaemia
- Sickle cell anaemia
- Pregnancy

Administration

The effective dosage of Gd-DTPA is 0.1 millimole (mmol) per kilogramme (kg) of body weight (mmol/kg), (approximately 0.2 ml/kg or 0.1 ml/lb), with a maximum dose of 20 ml. Gd-HP-DO3A has been approved for up to 0.3 mmol/kg or three times the dose of Gd-DTPA.

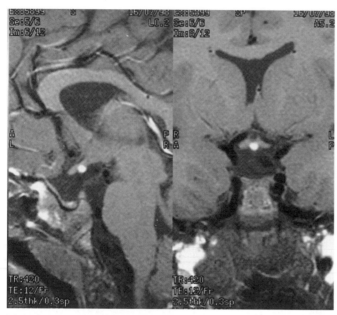

Fig. 42.3 Sagittal (left) and coronal (right) T1 weighted images after contrast showing an ectopic posterior pituitary.

Clinical applications (Fig. 42.3)

Gadolinium has proven invaluable in imaging the central nervous system because of its ability to pass through breakdowns in the blood–brain barrier (BBB). Clinical indications for gadolinium include:

- tumours pre and post surgery;
- pre and post radiotherapy;
- infection;
- infarction;
- inflammation;
- post-traumatic lesions;
- post operation lumbar disc;
- breast disease;
- prostatic disease;
- vessel patency and morphology (see Chapter 41).

Iron oxide

Iron oxides shorten relaxation times of nearby hydrogen atoms and therefore reduce the signal intensity in normal tissues. This results in a signal loss on proton density weighted or heavily T2 weighted images. Super-paramagnetic iron oxides are known as **T2 enhancement agents**. Iron oxide is taken up by the reticulo-endothelial system and excreted by the liver so that normal liver is dark and liver lesions are bright on T2 weighted images.

Side effects
- Mild to severe back, leg and groin pain is experienced and, in a few cases, head and neck pain.
- Patients experience digestive side-effects including nausea, vomiting and diarrohea.
- Anaphylactic-like reactions and hypotension have been reported in a few patients.

Contra-indications
- Contra-indicated in patients with known allergies / hypersensitivity to iron, parenteral dextran, parenteral iron-dextran or parenteral iron-polysaccaride preparations.
- Since the infusion is dark in colour, skin surrounding the infusion site might discolour if there is extraviscation.

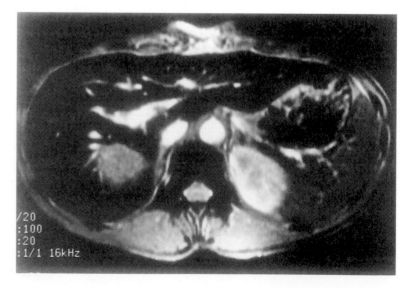

Fig. 42.4 This liver image was acquired with a fast T2 acquisition after an injection of a T2 shortening agent called Feridex©. Note that the normal portions of the liver are perfused by the agent and are black whereas the liver lesion remains somewhat unchanged by the iron oxide injection.

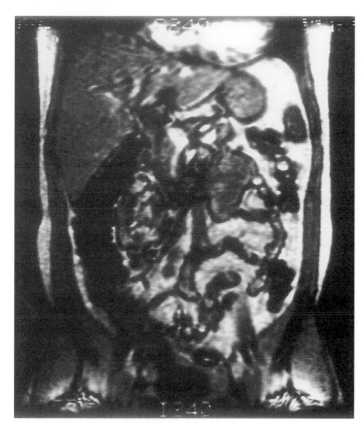

Fig. 42.5 Coronal image using an incoherent RF spoiled gradient echo sequence with dilute barium solution. Low signal intensity is demonstrated in the stomach.

Administration

The recommended dose of iron oxide is 0.56 mg of iron per kg of body weight. If using Feridex® dilute in 100 ml of 50% dextrose and give I.V. over 30 min. The diluted drug is administered through a 5 micron filter at a rate of 2–4 mmol/min. This agent should be used within 8 hours following dilution.

Clinical applications

This is mainly used in liver imaging where normal liver is dark on T2 weighted images and lesions appear bright (Fig. 42.4).

Other contrast agents

Gastro-intestinal contrast agents are sometimes used for bowel enhancement. These include barium (Fig. 42.5), ferromagnetic agents and fatty substances. However due to constant peristalsis, these agents enhance bowel motion artefacts more often than enhancing pathologic lesions. The use of anti-spasmodic agents helps to retard peristalsis to decrease these artefacts. Other agents include helium which is inhaled and assists in the evaluation of lung perfusion (Fig. 42.6).

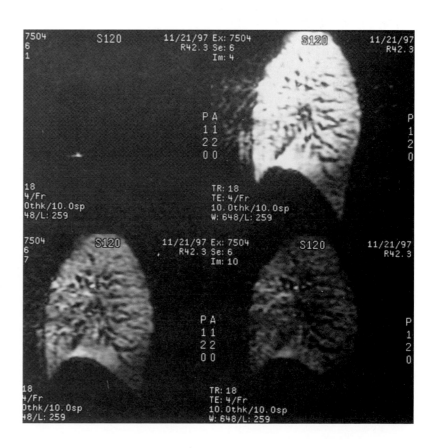

Fig. 42.6 Sagittal T1 weighted incoherent (spoiled) GRE sequences through the lung before (upper left), during (upper right) and after (lower left and right) inhalation of hyperpolarized helium.

Permanent magnets

Permanent magnets consist of ferromagnetic substances that have magnetic susceptibility greater than 1. They are easily magnetized and retain this magnetization (see Chapter 1). Examples of substances used are iron, cobalt and nickel. The most common material used is an alloy of aluminium, nickel and cobalt, known as **Alnico**.

Advantages

• They have open design; children, obese and claustrophobic patients are scanned with ease. Interventional and dynamic procedures are possible.
• They require no power supply and are therefore low in operating costs.
• The magnetic field created by a permanent magnet has lines of flux running vertically, keeping the magnetic field virtually confined within the boundaries of the scan room.

Disadvantages

• They are excessively heavy; only low fixed field-strengths (0.2–0.3 T) can be achieved.
• Longer scan times are needed, due to lower field strengths.

Electromagnets

Electromagnets utilize the laws of electromagnetic induction by passing an electrical current through a series of wires to produce a magnetic field (see Chapter 1). This physical phenomenon is utilized to produce RF coils and the static magnetic field.

Resistive magnets

The magnetic field strength in a resistive magnet is dependent upon the current that passes through its coils of wire. The direction of the main magnetic field in a resistive magnet follows the right-hand thumb rule and produces lines of flux running horizontally from the head to the foot of the magnet.

Advantages

• They are lighter in weight than permanent magnets.
• Capital costs are low.

Disadvantages

• The operational costs of the resistive magnet are quite high due to the large quantities of power required to maintain the magnetic field.
• The maximum field strength in a system of this type is less than 0.3 T due to its excessive power requirements. Therefore scan times are longer.
• The resistive system is relatively safe as the field can be turned off instantaneously. However, this type of magnet does create significant stray fringe magnetic fields.

Superconducting electromagnets

The resistance of the coils of wire is dependent upon the material of which the loops of wire are made, the length of the wire in the loop, the cross-sectional area of the wire and temperature. The latter can be controlled so that resistance is minimized.

As resistance decreases, the current dissipation also decreases. Therefore if the resistance is reduced, the energy required to maintain the magnetic field is decreased. As temperature decreases, resistance also decreases. As absolute zero of temperature (minus 273°C or 4°K) is approached, resistance is virtually absent, so that a high magnetic field can be maintained with no input power or driving voltage required. This is the basis of the function of the supercooled, superconducting magnet. The direction of the main magnetic field runs horizontally like that of the resistive system, from the head to the foot of the magnet.

Initially, current is passed through the loops of wire to create the magnetic field or bring the field up to strength (ramping). Then the wires are supercooled with substances known as cryogens (usually liquid helium [He] or liquid nitrogen [N]), to eliminate resistance. Since He and N are stable, they can be placed in a vacuum so that they do not rapidly boil off or return to their gaseous state. This is called a **cryogen bath** and it actually surrounds the coils of wire and is housed in the system between insulated vacuums.

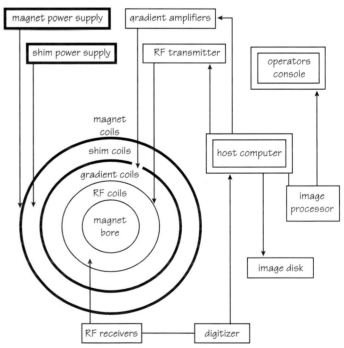

Fig. 43.1 Position of the magnet in a typical MR1 system.

Advantages

• It gives high magnetic field strengths (0.5–3 T) with low power requirements (after the magnetic field has been ramped up).
• There are low operating costs. With resistance virtually eliminated, there is no longer a mechanism to dissipate current, therefore no additional power input is required to maintain the high magnetic field strength.
• Advanced applications are possible and optimum image quality is obtained.

Disadvantages

• There is a high capital cost.
• Fringe fields are significant, so shielding is necessary.
• The tunnel design renders it unsuitable for large or claustrophobic patients. Interventional and dynamic studies are also difficult.

Shim coils

Owing to design limitations, it is almost impossible to create an electromagnet with coils of wire that are evenly spaced (equidistant from one end of the solenoid to the other). As the strength of the field is dependent on the distance between the loops, unevenly spaced loops create sags or **inhomogeneities** in the main magnetic field. These are measured in parts per million (ppm).

To correct for these inhomogeneities, another loop of current-carrying wire is placed in the area of the inhomogeneity. This, in effect, compensates for the sag in the main magnetic field and thus creates magnetic field homogeneity or evenness. This process is called **shimming** and the extra loop of wire is called a **shim** coil. For imaging purposes, homogeneity on the order of 10 ppm is required. Spectroscopic procedures require a more homogeneous environment of 1 ppm.

RF coils consist of loops of wire which, when a current is passed through them, produce a magnetic field at 90° to B_0.

Transmit coils

Energy is transmitted at the resonant frequency of hydrogen in the form of a short intense burst of radio frequency known as a radio-frequency pulse (see Chapter 4). The main magnetic field of a permanent magnet is usually vertical, whereas an electromagnet type of magnet has horizontal flux lines. Therefore the secondary field of the RF transmitter coil occurs in the horizontal axis in permanent magnets, and in the transverse or vertical axes in electromagnets magnets.

The main coils that transmit RF in most systems are:
• a body coil usually located within the bore of the magnet itself;
• a head coil.

The body coil is the main RF transmitter and transmits RF for most examinations excluding head imaging (when the head coil is used). The body and head coil are also capable of receiving RF, i.e. acting as receiver coils.

Receiver coils

RF coils placed in the transverse plane generate a voltage within them when a moving magnetic field cuts across the loops of wire. This voltage is the MR signal that is sampled to form an image. In order to induce an MR signal, the transverse magnetization must occur perpendicular to the receiver coils.

RF coil types

The configuration of the RF transmitter and receiver probes or coils directly affects the quality of the MR signal. There are several types of coil currently used in MR imaging: transmit/receive coils; surface coils and phased array coils.

Transmit/receive coils

A coil both transmits RF and receives the MR signal and is often called a **transceiver**. It encompasses the entire anatomy and can be used for either head or total body imaging. Head and body coils of a type known as the bird-cage configuration are used to image relatively large areas and yield uniform SNR over the entire imaging volume. However, even though the volume coils are responsible for uniform excitation over a large area, because of their large size they generally produce images with lower SNR than other types of coils. The signal quality produced by these coils has been significantly increased by a process known as **quadrature excitation and detection**.

Surface coils

Coils of this type are used to improve the SNR when imaging structures near the surface of the patient. Generally, the nearer the coil is situated to the structure under examination, the greater the SNR. This is because the coil is closer to the signal-emitting anatomy, and

only noise in the vicinity of the coil is received rather than over the entire body.

Surface coils are usually small and especially shaped so that they can be easily placed near the anatomy to be imaged with little or no discomfort to the patient. However, signal (and noise) is received only from the sensitive volume of the coil that corresponds to the area located around the coil. The size of this area extends to the circumference of the coil and at a depth into the patient equal to the radius of the coil. There is therefore a fall off of signal as the distance from the coil is increased in any direction.

Intra-cavity coils (such as rectal coils) or local coils, can be used to receive signal deep within the patient. As the SNR is enhanced when using local coils, greater spatial resolution of small structures can often be achieved. When using local coils, the body coil is used to transmit RF and the local coil is used to receive the MR signal.

Phased array coils

These consist of multiple coils and receivers whose individual signals are combined to create one image with improved SNR and increased coverage. Therefore the advantages of small surface coils (increased SNR and resolution), are combined with a large FOV for increased anatomy coverage. Usually up to four coils and receivers are grouped together either to increase longitudinal coverage or to improve uniformity across a whole volume. During data acquisition each individual coil receives signal from its own small usable FOV. The signal output from each coil is separately received and processed but

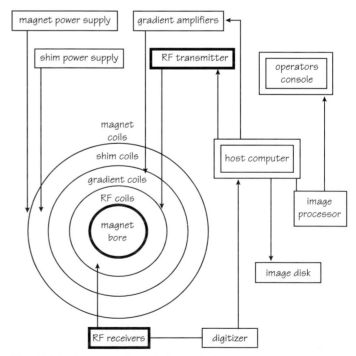

Fig. 44.1 Position of the RF coils in a typical MRI system.

then combined to form one single, larger FOV. As each coil has its own receiver the amount of noise received is limited to its small FOV, and all the data are acquired in a single sequence rather than four individual ones.

Large coil	Small coil
Large area of uniform signal reception	Small area of signal reception
Increased likelihood of aliasing with small FOV	Less likely to produce aliasing artefact
Positioning of patient not too critical	Positioning of coil critical
Lower SNR and resolution	High SNR and resolution

45 Gradients

Gradient coils provide a linear gradation or slope of the magnetic field strength from one end of the magnet to the other. This is achieved by passing current through the gradient coils (see Chapter 21).
- The direction of the current through the coil determines whether the magnetic field strength is increased or decreased relative to isocentre.
- The polarity of the current flowing through the coil determines which end of the gradient is higher than isocentre (positive) and which end is lower (negative).

Gradient coils are powered by **gradient amplifiers**. There are two gradient amplifiers for each gradient, one affixed to the high end of the gradient, the other to the low. Faults in the gradients or gradient amplifiers can result in geometric distortions in the MR image.

By varying the magnetic field strength, gradients provide position dependant variation of signal frequency and are therefore used for:
- slice selection;
- frequency encoding;
- phase encoding;
- rewinding (see Chapter 16);
- spoiling (see Chapter 17).

To apply a gradient, current is passed through a gradient coil. The change in field strength gradually increases to maximum dependent on the magnitude of the current. The gradient remains at maximum for a specific period of time and is then switched off. The change in field strength gradually decreases until there is no change, i.e. the magnetic field strength along the bore is equal to the main field strength of the magnet.

The **maximum amplitude** of a gradient is the maximum achievable change of field strength per metre along the bore of the magnet. This factor determines the maximum resolution possible because:
- steep slice select gradients are required for thin slices;
- steep phase encoding gradients are required for fine phase matrices;

- steep frequency encoding gradients are required for small fields of view.
- The **rise time** of a gradient is the time required to achieve the maximum amplitude.
- The **slew rate** is a function of rise time and amplitude. These factors determine the shortest scan times achievable.
- The **duty cycle** is the percentage of time the gradient is at maximum amplitude.

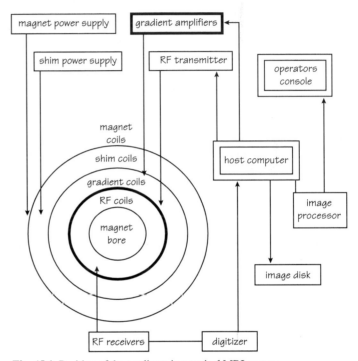

Fig. 45.1 Position of the gradients in a typical MRI system.

46 Other hardware

The pulse control unit

The pulse control unit is responsible for synchronizing the application of the gradients and RF pulses in a pulse sequence.

• Gradient coils are switched on and off very rapidly and at precise times during the pulse sequence.

• Gradient amplifiers supply the power to the gradient coils and a pulse control unit coordinates the functions of the gradient amplifiers and the coils so that they can be switched on and off at the appropriate times.

• For transmission and amplification of the RF, RF at the resonant frequency is transmitted by the RF transceiver, passes through frequency synthesisers to the RF amplifier and then through an RF monitor which ensures that safe levels of RF are delivered to the patient.

• The received RF signal from the coil is filtered, amplified and then passes to the array processor for Fast Fourier Transform. These data are then transmitted to the image processor so that each pixel can be allocated a grey scale colour in the image.

Operator interface

MRI computer systems vary with manufacturer. Most however consist of:

• a minicomputer with expansion capabilities;

• an array processor for Fourier transformation;

• an image processor that takes data from the array processor to form an image;

• hard disk drives for storage of raw data and pulse sequence parameters;

• a power distribution mechanism to distribute and filter the alternating current.

Data storage

For permanent storage of MR image data, data may be archived onto either magnetic tape or optical disks. This archive function can also be accessed through the operator's console. Images are stored so that cases can be retrieved for further manipulation and imaging in the future. They may also be used for comparison when repeat examinations are performed on the same patient.

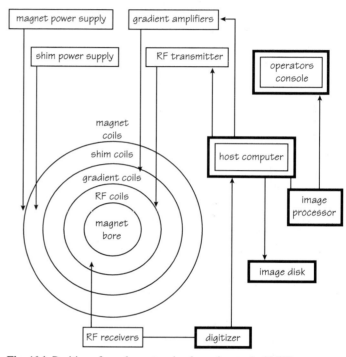

Fig. 46.1 Position of supplementary hardware in a typical MRI system.

47 Bioeffects

Static magnetic field-bioeffects

Current guidelines recommend a maximum limit of 2.5 T for clinical imaging rising to 3 T or 4 T for research purposes. Some small-bore systems are allowed to operate at higher field strengths.

The following points are *fundamentally* important with regard to the potentially harmful effects of the static magnetic field.

• The static field is always present (24 hours a day, 365 days a year to infinity). It is switched on even when the system is out of use.
• The fringe field may extend several metres beyond the examination room and therefore any harmful effects or risks may come into play at some distance from the scanner.

There is no conclusive evidence for irreversible or harmful bioeffects in humans below 2.5 T. Reversible abnormalities may include:

• an increase in the amplitude of the T-wave that can be noted on an ECG due to the magnetic hydrodynamic effect (also known as the magnetic haemodynamic effect);
• heating of patients;
• fatigue;
• headaches;
• hypotension;
• irritability.

Time-varying field bioeffects

Gradients create a time-varying magnetic field. This changing field occurs during the scanning sequence. It is not present at other times and therefore exposure is restricted to patients and to relatives who may be present in the scan room during the examination.

The health consequences are not related to the strength of the gradient field, but to changes in the magnetic field that cause induced currents. Nerves, blood vessels and muscles that act as conductors in the body, may be affected. The induced current is greater in peripheral tissues since the amplitude of the gradient is higher away from magnetic isocentre.

Time-varying bioeffects from gradient coils include:

• light flashes in the eyes;
• alterations in the biochemistry of cells and fracture union;

• mild cutaneous sensations;
• involuntary muscle contractions;
• cardiac arrhythmias.

RF transmit coils also produce time-varying fields. The predominant biological effect of RF irradiation absorption is the potential heating of tissue. As an excitation pulse is applied, some nuclei absorb the RF energy and enter the high energy state. As they relax, nuclei give off this absorbed energy to the surrounding lattice. As excitation frequency is increased, absorbed energy is also increased, therefore heating of tissue is largely frequency dependent.

Energy dissipation can be described in terms of **specific absorption rate (SAR)**. SAR is expressed in watts/kg, a quantity that depends on:

• the induced electric field;
• the pulse duty cycle;
• the tissue density;
• the conductivity;
• the patient's size.

SAR is used to calculate an expected increase in body temperature during an average examination. In the UK, it is recommended that this should not exceed 1 °C during the examination.

Studies show that patient exposure up to three times the recommended levels produces no serious adverse effects, despite elevations in skin and body temperatures. As body temperature increases, blood pressure and heart rate also increase slightly. Even though these effects seem insignificant, patients with compromised thermo-regulatory systems may not be candidates for MR.

Radio frequency fields can be responsible for significant burn hazards due to electrical currents that are produced in conductive loops. Equipment used in MRI such as ECG leads and surface coils, should therefore be used with extreme caution. When using a surface coil, the operator must be careful to prevent any electrically conductive material (i.e. cable of surface coil) from forming a 'conductive loop' with itself or with the patient.

Table 47.1 Recommended restricted levels of exposure to static magnetic field – patients, staff and volunteers.

	Lower static fields	Higher static fields
Whole body	2.5 T	4 T
Limbs	4 T	4 T

Table 47.2 Recommended exposure restriction on whole body SAR (time, t, is in minutes).

Duration of exposure (min)	Lower level SAR (W/kg)	Higher level SAR (W/kg)
$30 < t$	1	2
$15 < t > 30$	$30/t$	$60/t$
$t < 15$	2	4

48 Projectiles

The projectile effect of a metal object exposed to the field can seriously compromise the safety of anyone sited between the object and the magnet system. **The potential harm cannot be over emphasized.** Even small objects, such as paper clips and hair pins, have a terminal velocity of 40 mph when pulled into a 1.5 T magnet, and therefore pose a serious risk to the patient and anyone else present in the scan room. Larger objects such as scissors travel at much higher velocities and may be fatal to any person standing in their path.

Many types of clinical equipment are ferromagnetic and should never be brought into the scan room. These include:

- surgical tools;
- scissors;
- clamps;
- oxygen tanks.

Metallic implants and prosthesis

These produce serious effects which include: torque or twisting in the field, heating effects and artefacts on MR images. The type of metal used in such implants is one factor that determines the force exerted on them in magnetic fields. While non-ferrous metallic implants may show little or no deflection to the field, they could cause significant heating due to their inability to dissipate the heat caused by radio-frequency absorption.

Intra-cranial aneurysm clips

Clip motion may damage the vessel, resulting in haemorrhage, ischaemia or death. Currently, many intra-cranial clips are made of a non-ferromagnetic substance such as titanium. However recent studies have indicated that even these may deflect in a magnetic field. It is therefore recommended that imaging of patients with aneurysm clips is delayed until the type of clip is emphatically identified as non-ferrous and non-deflectable.

Cardiac pacemakers

Even field strengths as low as 10 G may be sufficient to cause deflection, programming changes, and closure of the reed switch that converts a pacemaker to an asynchronous mode. In addition, patients who have had their pacemaker removed may have pacer wires left within the body that could act as an antenna, and (by induced currents) cause cardiac fibrillation.

Prosthetic heart valves

Considerably deflected by the static magnetic field. The deflection however is minimal compared with normal pulsatile cardiac motion. Therefore, although patients with most valvular implants are considered safe for MR, as there are valves whose integrity is compromised, careful screening for valve type is advised.

Cochlear implants

These are attracted to the magnetic field and are magnetically or electronically activated.

Intra-ocular ferrous foreign bodies

It is not uncommon for patients who have worked with sheet metal to have metal fragments or slivers located in and around the eye. Since the magnetic field exerts a force on ferromagnetic objects, a metal fragment in the eye could move or be displaced and cause injury to the eye or surrounding tissue. Therefore all patients with a suspected eye injury must be X-rayed before the MR examination.

Orthopaedic implants

Most orthopaedic implants show no deflection within the main magnetic field. However a large metallic implant, such as a hip prosthesis, can become heated by currents induced in the metal by the magnetic and radio frequency fields. It appears, however, that such heating is relatively low. The majority of orthopaedic implants have been imaged with MR without incident.

Abdominal surgical clips

These are generally safe for MR because they become anchored by fibrous tissue but produce artefacts in proportion to their size and can distort the image.

49 Screening and safety procedures

Owing to the hazards particularly associated with projectiles, all persons entering the controlled area must satisfy a safety screening procedure. It is also recommended that all objects are tested with a hand-held bar magnet before entering the MR scan room. In addition, it is advised that all nursing, housekeeping, fire department, emergency and MR personnel are educated about the potential risks and hazards of the static magnetic field. Signs should be attached at all entrances to the magnetic field (including the fringe field) to deter entry into the scan room with ferromagnetic objects.

Screening procedure

Two distinct safety zones may be identified around the MR system: the exclusion zone and the security zone.

The exclusion zone

This is defined by the boundary of the 5 gauss line. A warning sign should be posted at all points of access to the exclusion zone. Entrance must be restricted to those people who have passed the screening procedure. In modern scanners the 5 G line is usually within the exclusion zone.

The security zone

An area (usually the magnet room itself) where the potential to cause projectile injuries exists due to the attraction of loose objects into the magnet.

Security zone precautions

• Have only one point of access, marked by a warning sign. People entering the scan room must be screened for any loose ferromagnetic objects prior to entry.
• The scan room door should be kept closed at all times when not in use.
• Patients must not be left unattended within the magnet room.
Several measures must be taken to ensure that no person approaches the magnetic field which could pose a risk either to themselves or to patients.
• There must be at least two physical barriers between the 5 G line and general public access. Lockable or magnetically switched doors and gates are preferable. Every barrier must clearly display a sign warning of the presence of a strong magnetic field with a list of devices that must not go beyond this point (e.g. pacemakers). These barriers and signs must be displayed 24 hours a day.
• There must be thorough screening of **any** person who is to enter the field. This includes radiographers, doctors, patients, relatives, cleaners and porters. No one is excluded.

All centres should have a proper screening policy that includes checking for:
• pacemakers;
• intra-ocular foreign bodies;
• metal devices or prostheses;
• cochlear implants;
• possibility of early pregnancy.

Most facilities provide a screening form that patients, relatives and other persons fill in before entering the magnetic field. This ensures that important questions have been addressed, and provides a record that screening has taken place. This may be very critical if an accident subsequently occurs.

Items such as watches, credit cards, money, pens and any other loose items must be removed before entering the magnetic field. Unremovable items such as splints must be thoroughly checked for safety with a hand-held bar magnet before entering the MR scan room.

Staff safety

Permanent personnel such as radiographers, radiologists and clerical staff need only complete a safety questionnaire at their first visit to the unit. Other staff such as visiting doctors or nurses accompanying patients must complete a safety form and remove all loose items at each visit if they are entering the magnetic field.

In shielded magnets, radiographic and radiological staff are not usually exposed to the static magnetic field when in the control room. However in unshielded, high field strength facilities, scanning personnel may permanently sit in a magnetic field of 30 G or more. There is no evidence to suggest that this is harmful in any way. Exposure to gradient and radio-frequency fields only occurs during the scan sequence and therefore staff are not usually subjected to it. However there are occasions when staff are required to be present in the room during the sequence. These include:

Table 49.1 Devices affected by the static field.

1 gauss	nuclear cameras
	PET scanners
	cyclotrons
	linear accelerators
	CT scanners
	ultrasound equipment
3 gauss	metal detector
	road traffic
	passenger and freight elevators
	power transformers
5 gauss	cardiac pacemakers
	neuro stimulators
	bio stimulation devices
10 gauss	computers
	water chiller
	emergency generators
	air conditioning chillers
	image processor
	disk drives
	magnetic tapes/
	floppy disks
	credit cards
	watches
30 gauss	remote console
50 gauss	operator console

- for patient reassurance;
- during dynamic imaging where contrast media is injected during the sequence;
- general anesthesia or sedation situations where patients must be carefully monitored;
- during interventional procedures such as biopsies.

Whilst a patient is only exposed to these fields for the short duration of the examination, staff under these circumstances may be subjected to repeated exposures. The potential harmful effects of these conditions have not yet been fully evaluated but at present some exposure to changing fields on an occasional basis is not thought to be harmful.

Pregnancy

As yet, there are no known biological effects of MRI on fetuses. However, there are a number of mechanisms that could potentially cause adverse effects as a result of the interaction of electromagnetic fields with developing fetuses. Cells undergoing division, which occurs during the first trimester of pregnancy, are more susceptible to these effects.

As yet, official guidelines have not been established, and so MR is neither recommended nor forbidden. In light of the high risk potential for pregnant patients in general, it has been suggested that any examination of pregnant patients should be delayed until the first trimester and then a written consent form should be signed by the patient before the examination.

MR facilities have established individual guidelines for pregnant employees in the magnetic resonance environment. The majority of units have determined that pregnant employees can safely enter the scan room, but leave while the RF and gradient fields are employed. Some facilities, however, recommend that the employee stay out of the magnetic field entirely during the first trimester of pregnancy.

50 Emergencies in the MR environment

Quenching

Quenching is the process whereby there is a sudden loss of absolute zero of temperature in the magnet coils so that they cease to be superconducting and become resistive. This results in helium escaping from the cryogen bath extremely rapidly. It may happen accidentally or can be manually instigated in the case of an emergency. Quenching may cause severe and irreparable damage to the superconducting coils, and so a manual quench should only be performed if a person is pinned to the magnet by a large metal object that cannot be removed by hand.

All systems should have helium venting equipment which removes the helium to the outside environment in the event of a quench. However, if this fails, helium vents into the room and replaces oxygen. For this reason, all scan rooms should contain an oxygen monitor that sounds an alarm if the oxygen falls below a certain level.

In the case of a quench

- Do not panic.
- Turn on scan room exhaust fan (if not automatically turned on by the oxygen monitor).
- Prop open door between operator room and hallway.
- Using the intercom, ask the patient to stay calm and remain on the table. Tell him/her that someone will be in shortly to offer assistance.
- Open window to scan room if so constructed.
- Prop open the door to the scan room.
- Enter the scan room, undock the table, help patient exit the scan room.
- Evacuate the area, returning when the air is restored to normal.

If helium is venting into the room, the scan room door may not open

- Try opening the scan room door several times. If the door cannot be opened after 45 seconds, open, or if necessary, break the window to the scan room to relieve the pressure.
- Enter the scan room through the door. If the door does not open, go through the window.
- Evacuate the patient as instructed above.

Magnetic field emergency

If someone is pinned against the magnet by a ferromagnetic object, or if some other magnetic-field-related emergency occurs, quench the magnet. A magnet quench will result in several days' downtime, so do not press the button except in a true emergency. Do not attempt to test this button; it should be tested only by qualified service personnel.

Patient emergency

Patients with the following conditions are at greatest risk for complications during MR scanning:

- likely to develop seizure or claustrophobic reaction;
- greater than normal potential for cardiac arrest;
- unconscious, heavily sedated or confused patients with whom no reliable communication can be maintained.

Since direct observation from the MR operator console is usually partially obscured by the magnet enclosure, be sure to monitor these patients closely at all times to identify quickly and respond to medical emergencies. In some cases, emergency personnel should remain with the patient or be on stand-by alert to help prevent serious complications or death.

If the patient needs emergency medical attention during the scanning session, follow the following procedure.

- Hit the Emergency Stop button on the console or magnet enclosure to abort the scan. Notify emergency personnel if necessary. Since ferromagnetic life-support and related equipment cannot be brought into the scan room, the patient must be evacuated.
- Evacuate the patient from the scan room as quickly as possible to a designated emergency medical treatment area outside the exclusion zone.
- Close the magnet door.
- Follow hospital emergency protocol.

Appendix

Table A.1 Artefacts and their remedies.

Artefacts	Axis	Remedy	Penalty
Truncation	phase	increase phase encodings	increase scan time
Phase mismapping	phase	respiratory compensation	may lose a slice
		swap phase and frequency	may need no phase wrap
		gating	variable TR variable image contrast increased scan time
		pre-saturation	may lose a slice
		gradient moment rephasing	increases minimum TE
Chemical shift	frequency	increase bandwidth	decrease minimum TE available decrease SNR
		reduce FOV	reduces SNR decreases resolution
		use chemical saturation	reduces SNR may lose slices
Chemical misregistration	phase	select TE at periodicity of fat and water	may lose a slice if TE is increased significantly
Aliasing	frequency and phase	no frequency wrap	none
		no phase wrap	may reduce SNR may increase scan time with some vendors increases motion artefact due to reduced NEX
		enlarge the FOV	reduces resolution
Zipper	frequency	call engineer	irate engineer!
Magnetic susceptibility	frequency and phase	use spin echo	not flow sensitive blood product may be missed
		remove metal where possible	none
Shading	frequency and phase	check shim load coil correctly prescan correctly	none
Motion	phase	use anti-spasmodics	costly, invasive
		immobilize patient	none
		counselling of patient all remedies for mismapping	none see previous
		sedation	possible side effects invasive, costly requires monitoring
Cross talk	slice select	none	none
Cross excitation	slice select	interleaving	doubles the scan time
		squaring off RF pulses	reduces SNR

Table A.2 A comparison of the acronyms used by manufacturers.

	GE	Philips	Siemens	Picker	Elscint	Hitachi	Shimadzu
Spin echo	MEMP VEMP	spin echo	spin echo	spin echo	spin echo	spin echo	spin echo
Fast spin echo	FSE	TSE	TSE	FSE		FSE	
Coherent gradient echo	GRASS	FFE	FISP	FAST	F short	GFEC	SSFP
Incoherent gradient echo (RF spoiled)	SPGR	T1 FFE		RF spoiled FAST			STAGE T1W
Incoherent gradient echo (gradient spoiled)	MPGR		FLASH		short	GRE	STAGE
Steady state free precession	SSFP	T2 FFE	PSIF	CE FAST	E short	GFEC contrast	STERF
Inversion recovery	MPIR	IR	IR	IR	IR	IR	IR
Short T1 inversion recovery	STIR	SPIR	STIR	STIR	STIR	STIR	STIR
Ultra fast	fast GRASS SPGR (IR/DE prep)	TFE	Turbo FLASH 3D MP RAGE	RAM FAST			SMASH
Pre-saturation	SAT	REST	SAT	pre-SAT	spatial pre-sat	SAT	SAT
Gradient moment rephasing	flow comp	FLAG	GMR	MAST	STILL	GR	SMART
Resp. compensation	resp. comp	PEAR	resp. trigger	resp. gating PRIZE	FREEZE	phase re-ordering	
Signal averaging	NEX	NSA	AC	NSA		NSA	
Partial averaging	fractional NEX	half scan	half Fourier	phase conjugate symmetry	single side encoding	half Fourier	
Partial echo	fractional echo	partial echo		read conjugate symmetry	single side view		
No phase wrap	no phase wrap	fold over suppression	over sampling	over sampling	anti aliasing	anti wrap	
Rectangular FOV	rect FOV	rect FOV	half Fourier imaging	under sampling	rect FOV	rect FOV	

Abbreviations used in Table A.2.

3D MP RAGE	3D magnetization prepared rapid gradient echo	MPGR	Multi planar gradient recalled acquisition in the steady state
AC	Number of acquisitions	MPIR	Multi planar inversion recovery
CE FAST	Contrast enhanced FAST	NEX	Number of excitations
DE prep	Driven equilibrium magnetization preparation	NSA	Number of signal averages
		PEAR	Phase encoding artefact reduction
E short	Short repetition technique based on echo	PSIF	Mirrored FISP
FAST	Fourier acquired steady state technique	RAM FAST	Rapid acquisition matrix FAST
		REST	Regional saturation technique
FFE	Fast field echo	RF spoiled FAST	RF spoiled Fourier acquired steady state
FISP	Fast imaging with steady precession	Short	Short repetition techniques
FLAG	Flow adjusted gradients	SMART	Shimadzu motion artefact reduction technique
FLASH	Fast low angled shot	SMASH	Short minimum angled shot
FREEZE	Respiratory selection of phase encoding steps	SPGR	Spoiled gradient recalled acquisition in the steady state
FSE	Fast spin echo	SPIR	Spectrally selective inversion recovery
F short	Short repetition technique based on free induction decay		
		SSFP	Steady state free precession
GFE	Gradient field echo	STAGE	Small tip angle gradient echo
GFEC	Gradient field echo with contrast	STERF	Steady state technique with refocused FID
GMR	Gradient moment rephasing		
GR	Gradient rephasing	STILL	Flow motion compensation
GRASS	Gradient recalled acquisition in the steady state	STIR	Short T1 inversion recovery
		TFE	Turbo field echo
IR prep	Inversion recovery magnetisation preparation	TSE	Turbo spin echo
		Turbo FLASH	Magnetization prepared sub second imaging technique
MAST	Motion artefact suppression		
MEMP	Multi echo multi planar	VEMP	Variable echo multi planar

Index

Page numbers in *italics* refer to figures; those in **bold** to tables. The alphabetical arrangement is letter-by-letter.

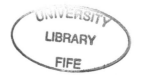